For
Orange Mummy

Contents

Preface

A joint working party of the Royal College of Obstetricians and Gynaecologists (RCOG) and the Royal College of Midwives (RCM) called for referenced, evidence-based, multidisciplinary policies for the management of all key conditions and situations on the delivery suite, and it is a requirement for Clinical Negligence Scheme for Trusts (CNST) accreditation that maternity units have these. This book originates from the guidelines I put together for the delivery suite at the Royal Oldham Hospital.

The primary purpose of a delivery-suite handbook is to ensure that standard practice is maintained and not to discuss theory or teach skills. A handbook is more about what to do and when, and less about how to do it. The theoretical principles and descriptions of how to perform various procedures are to be found in the appropriate midwifery and obstetric textbooks.

Delivery-suite guidelines should not read like textbooks. In writing new guidelines for Oldham, a pragmatic approach was adopted. The size was changed from A4 to C5 to make it a handbook in every sense. The format was changed so that there was less prose and more bullet points and tick boxes. References have been excluded from the main text, and pooled at the end of each section under 'Further reading'. The layout is designed to be user-friendly. Throughout this book there has been a focus on managing risk. The tick boxes allow copies of the relevant pages to be photocopied and inserted into the woman's hospital records, with the boxes ticked as a supplementary record of the woman's care in labour.

Although these guidelines were written originally for one hospital, they are readily adaptable to local needs elsewhere. Any Trust wishing to adapt these guidelines is welcome to do so, but please inform the publisher. This handbook will also be useful to training-grade doctors for on-the-job learning and in preparation for college examinations.

Doctors and midwives constitute a team and have responsibilities to the mother and to each other. Also, normal and abnormal labour are a continuum. It is hoped that these guidelines will facilitate a unified approach to patient care.

Leroy Edozien

Acknowledgements

This book is a compendium of best practice distilled from research publications, textbooks, the *Cochrane Library*, guidelines produced by the RCOG, the Confidential Enquiries into Maternal Deaths, and labour-ward protocols of a number of hospitals, with embellishment from the author's personal experience.

Section 2 (Normal and low-risk labour) draws from guidelines written originally for the Royal Oldham Hospital by senior midwives Viv Dickinson and Bev Wilkinson. The chapter on epidural analgesia is informed by guidelines written for Oldham by Dr Ian Brocklehurst, Consultant Anaesthetist. Dr Ross Macnab, Consultant Anaesthetist, Manchester, kindly provided material for and commented on the chapters dealing with epidural analgesia, recovery of the obstetric patient and high-dependency care. The chapter on care of the woman in labour with a pre-viable fetus is based on guidelines written by Sue Brierley, Midwifery Sister, Oldham. Dr Ngozi Edi-Osagie, Consultant Neonatologist, Manchester, edited the chapter on neonatal resuscitation.

Midwifery, anaesthetic, paediatric and obstetric staff on the delivery suite in Oldham also submitted comments and corrections when the first version of this book was piloted. Professor Philip J Steer, Chelsea and Westminster Hospital, made invaluable comments that informed the final version.

I am indebted to Peter Richardson, Managing Director of RSM Press Limited; but for his faith, this book may never have been published. I have been privileged to have an efficient, creative and personable editor at the RSM Press, Natalie Baderman. The book has been enriched by the comments and queries of the copy editor.

The contributions of all are acknowledged gratefully.

Foreword

In these days of clinical governance, all maternity units should have guidelines. But guidelines are not easy to write. They take a great deal of time, effort, and careful thought. Leroy Edozien has performed a great service in making his guidelines available to a wide readership. As he points out, this is not a textbook. It is not even an exhaustive list of all the various options for managing any particular clinical situation. It is, however, a careful description of at least one way, consistent with current acceptable clinical practice, of dealing with all the common problems that occur on labour wards. The logistics that he lays out are those needed for the practical organization of care, an aspect that is often missing in traditional textbooks.

It is important to appreciate that guidelines are just that – they are not prescriptive in all circumstances. Where there is evidence, the guidelines in this book reflect it. When, through lack of evidence, they have of necessity to be opinion-based, then sometimes they diverge from those I personally follow. But they are always reasonable, and medico-legally defensible. This is a vital safeguard for the inexperienced, until they develop enough knowledge to form their own opinions. The guidelines may not all be suitable for all units, because local needs vary. However, they will be invaluable as a template for developing guidelines appropriate to each individual unit, and as a curriculum on which to build clinical skills training. Knowledge grows and views change, and so it is ideal that all units should have their own guidelines development committee to review and update guidelines regularly. However, building from scratch a comprehensive set of guidelines such as are contained in this volume can take years rather than weeks. Accordingly, the author has generously suggested that anyone is welcome to adopt and adapt these guidelines, as long as they inform the publisher. They could even be the basis for developing a set of guidelines on your local intranet, an approach that we use at the Chelsea and Westminster Hospital because it makes updating easier and less expensive. One needs to be aware that knowledge is an organic, developing thing, and, like plants, guidelines that fail to grow and develop continuously will die. This book contains many seeds that, when planted in your own practice, will flourish, and for anyone interested in growing their own clinical governance framework, it should be cultivated. Fed new information, and occasionally pruned, it will grow into something even more valuable than it is today.

Philip J Steer

Abbreviations

ALT	alanine aminotransferase
APH	antepartum haemorrhage
APTT	activated partial thromboplastin time
ARDS	adult respiratory distress syndrome
ARM	artificial rupture of fetal membranes
bd	twice daily
BLS	basic life support
BP	blood pressure
CNST	Clinical Negligence Scheme for Trusts
CPR	cardiopulmonary resuscitation
CRP	C-reactive protein
CS	caesarean section
CSF	cerebrospinal fluid
CTG	cardiotocograph
CVP	central venous pressure
DIC	disseminated intravascular coagulopathy
DVT	deep venous thrombosis
ECG	electrocardiography
ECV	external cephalic version
EUA	examination under anaesthetic
FBC	full blood count
FBS	fetal blood sampling
FDP	fibrin degradation products
FFP	fresh frozen plasma
FISH	fluorescent *in situ* hybridization
FSE	fetal scalp electrodes
GBS	group B haemolytic streptococci
[Hb]	haemoglobin concentration
HDU	high-dependency unit
HELLP	haemolysis, elevated liver enzymes, low platelets
HVS	high vaginal swab
IM (or im)	intramuscular
ITU	intensive therapy unit
IUGR	intrauterine growth restriction
IV (or iv)	intravenous
IVH	intraventricular haemorrhage
LFT	liver function tests
LMWH	low-molecular weight heparin

MAP	mean arterial pressure
NSAID	nonsteroidal anti-inflammatory drug
NTD	neural tube defect
ODA	operating department assistant
OP	occipitoposterior
PDS	polydioxanone sulphate sutures
PPH	postpartum haemorrhage
PROM	prelabour rupture of membranes
PT	prothrombin time
pv	per vaginum
qds	four times daily
RCM	Royal College of Midwives
RCOG	Royal College of Obstetricians and Gynaecologists
RDS	respiratory distress syndrome
Rh	Rhesus
SC (or sc)	subcutaneous
SCBU	special-care baby unit
SHO	senior house officer
SROM	spontaneous rupture of fetal membranes
tds	three times daily
TED	thromboembolism-deterrent stockings
U/E	urea and electrolytes
VE	vaginal examination
V/Q	ventilation–perfusion scan
VTE	venous thromboembolism

Section 1: Approach to care

'... a shift in attention from what is done to patients to what is accomplished for them'

    – Committee on Quality of Healthcare in America. Institute of Medicine, *Crossing the Quality Chasm: A New Health System for the 21st Century*. Washington, DC: National Academy Press, 2001, p. 44

Bleep/crash calls

Bleeps

Obstetric SHO: ......

Obstetric registrar: ......

Paediatric SHO: ......

Paediatric registrar: ......

Anaesthetic registrar: ......

Anaesthetic assistant: ......

Emergencies

Crash calls for obstetric, paediatric and anaesthetic SHO and registrar:

Obstetrics: ......

Ask for appropriate doctor to be bleeped urgently. State the place (eg delivery suite and room no.).

Paediatrics: ......

Request the second on paediatrician urgently. State the place (eg delivery suite and room no.).

Anaesthetics: ......

State the place (eg delivery suite).

NB: If more than one of the specialties is required, it is not necessary to make more than one call. Bleep ...... and ask for an urgent call to go out to the appropriate specialties. State the place (eg delivery suite and room no.).

Cardiac arrest: ......

State the place (eg delivery suite and room no.).

Fire: Activate the fire alarm. Dial ......

Wait for call to be acknowledged. Proceed appropriately with fire drill, as instructed at the annual fire lecture.

Communication

For efficient delivery of care, it is important that lines of communication are well defined. The consultant under whose care the mother is booked is ultimately responsible for her care. For each shift on the delivery suite, one midwife of grade G or above will be designated team leader (or coordinator) and will be responsible for coordinating the work of the delivery suite, providing necessary support, guidance and supervision of midwives and medical staff. The team leader should be informed regularly of each mother's progress. Names of the lead midwife and the obstetric, anaesthetic and paediatric medical staff on duty will be written on the designated notice board.

All members of the duty obstetric team should ensure that they are readily accessible and available at all times.

The lines of communication for the midwife are through the team leader or senior midwife on duty and the resident medical staff. However, any midwife or other member of staff who has concerns about a woman's care may contact the registrar or consultant (obstetric or anaesthetic) directly.

If a non-duty consultant has an interest in the management of a particular patient, then this should be marked clearly in the case notes; the senior midwife or registrar will need to contact this consultant when the woman is admitted and if problems arise afterwards.

All high-risk patients admitted to the labour ward must be seen by the SHO or registrar as soon as possible.

There should be a personal handover of patient care at the shift/on-call changeover of both midwifery and medical staff. There should be ward rounds at 0830, 1300 and 1700 and a telephone review with the consultant at 2200.

The registrar should be informed immediately of any untoward problems and of any of the following conditions (but note that this is not an exhaustive list):

- antepartum haemorrhage
- postpartum haemorrhage
- malpresentation
- cord prolapse/cord presentation
- severe pre-eclampsia/eclampsia
- multiple pregnancy
- preterm labour
- prelabour rupture of membranes

- abnormal fetal heart rate
- any pregnancy identified as high-risk in the case notes
- diabetes mellitus
- cardiac disease
- intrauterine death
- large baby
- previous caesarean section.

If there is any delay in response in cases such as prolapsed cord or if the registrar is unavailable due to another emergency, then the consultant on call should be called immediately.

For women at high risk, a plan of management should be made antenatally and written in the handheld and hospital records, with a clear signature. Early identification of risk factors, anticipation of problems, and effective communication are key factors for good management.

In anticipation of events, the anaesthetist should be informed at an early stage of any of the following:

- antepartum haemorrhage
- twin pregnancy in labour
- breech vaginal delivery
- previous caesarean section
- woman at risk of postpartum haemorrhage
- pre-eclampsia
- obese patient who may require operative intervention
- medical conditions such as diabetes, sickle cell and heart disease
- history of anaphylaxis.

'Anaesthetists responsible for obstetric services should liaise with midwives, obstetricians and physicians to agree management for successful delivery. The anaesthetist must become involved in the management of the "at risk" patient at an early stage ...'

> – Hibbard BM, Anderson MM, Drife JO, *et al. Report on Confidential Enquiries into Maternal Deaths in the United Kingdom 1991–1993.* London: HMSO, 1996, Chapter 9 p. 101

'Obstetricians failed to give adequate warning of impending problems to anaesthetic departments in at least six of the maternal deaths in this triennium. The lack of consultation with anaesthetic colleagues contributed significantly to a number of these deaths.'

> – Thomas TA, Cooper GM. Anaesthesia. In: Lewis G (ed). *Why Mothers Die, 1997–1999. The Fifth Report of the Confidential Enquiries into Maternal Deaths in the United Kingdom.* London: RCOG Press, 2001, p. 139

Documentation

All records should be written in black ink and handwriting must be legible.

Care given should be documented carefully and thoughtfully. All examinations, results, clinical communications and maternal requests should be documented accurately on the labour notes, partogram and CTG trace as appropriate.

All entries to the records must be clearly signed, dated and timed (use 24-hour clock). Illegible signatures are not acceptable. Always print your name and grade below your signature.

Use abbreviations sparingly, and only those listed on pp. xii–xiii.

Every loose-leaf sheet in the notes must have patient identification. The responsibility for this rests with the first person that writes on that page.

Consent for examination, CS and other interventions must follow standard policy (see Appendix 1, pp. 227–230).

Every operative delivery should be written up in detail, with the date, time, indication(s), findings and any complications stated clearly.

The time of decision to perform a CS, and the degree of urgency (see p. 72), should be documented. The time of commencement of CS, ie 'knife to skin', should be recorded in the swab book.

Before filing any results, check that they belong to the correct patient, annotate any action required or taken, and append your signature.

Every CTG trace should bear the patient's identification label and the date and time of commencement and completion. Maternal pulse should be recorded regularly on the trace, along with any key events in care. Any loss of contact or discontinuation should be annotated on the trace.

Sign and date all CTGs, and file them securely with the clinical records.

The standard setting of 1 cm/min should not be altered on the CTG monitor.

Never try to alter existing notes. If corrections are necessary, draw a line through the incorrect entry and sign and date the additional note.

All midwifery records must comply with Midwives Rule 42 (see Further reading, p. 15).

The statutory limitation on obstetric litigation is not until the child is 21 years of age, so notes relating to pregnancy care must be maintained intact for this duration.

Admission to, and discharge home from, delivery suite

Admission

The initial assessment will be by a named midwife to whom the woman has been introduced. Where indicated (see Communication, pp. 4–5), the admitting midwife should refer to the SHO or registrar on duty, without delay. The antenatal clinic records and records of any admissions in the pregnancy should be reviewed and any special instructions noted. A plan of care should be devised with the woman, building on wishes and plans agreed during antenatal care. This plan should be flexible, subject to review during labour. Document the reason for admission, the findings on assessment and the plan of care.

Discharge

An experienced midwife may discharge a woman home when labour has been excluded, provided the following criteria are met:

☐ Normal, uneventful pregnancy at 37–40 weeks.
☐ Normal medical history.
☐ Normal maternal observations.
☐ Normal/reactive admission CTG, where this test is indicated.
☐ No abnormal vaginal loss.
☐ Normal vaginal examination with no indication that labour has established.
☐ Intact membranes.
☐ First referral to delivery suite.
☐ Woman is happy to go home.
☐ Follow-up appointment is given.

A woman who presents with deviations from the above criteria should be referred to the SHO/registrar on call for further assessment. A woman not wishing to go home may be transferred to the antenatal ward.

Clinical incident reporting

Aims

This guidance aims to:

- promote the improvement of quality in patient care
- enhance patient safety
- set out the directorate's approach to the reporting of clinical incidents in obstetrics;
- ensure compliance with
  - the Trust's risk management strategy
  - the Trust's clinical incident policy
  - CNST clinical risk standards
  - recommendations in *An Organisation with a Memory* (see Further reading, p. 15).

What is a clinical incident?

A clinical incident is an incident or accident that happened to a patient during or as a result of treatment or care and that has caused, or could cause, an adverse outcome.

All incidents on the trigger list, and any other that, in the opinion of the ward manager, falls within the scope of this definition, must be reported as detailed below.

It is not practicable to provide an exhaustive list of clinical incidents, but the more common examples are:

- maternal death
- stillbirth
- neonatal death
- low Apgar score: <6 at 5 minutes
- undiagnosed breech
- shoulder dystocia
- major postpartum haemorrhage (≥1000 ml)
- postpartum [Hb] <8 g/dl
- eclampsia or other fits
- unexpected transfer to neonatal unit, including neonatal seizures
- drug errors
- significant infections
- loss of clinical materials, eg swabs

- unavailability of health record
- return to theatre
- third- and fourth-degree tears
- readmission of either mother or baby
- unavailability of any facility or equipment, including neonatal unit cots
- misdiagnosis of antenatal screening tests
- unplanned home birth
- cord pH <7.0
- maternal transfer to ITU
- maternal resuscitation
- trauma to bladder or other organs
- first stage of labour >17 hours
- second stage of labour >3 hours
- birth injury
  - subdural haematoma or tear of falx cerebri
  - any fracture, eg skull, clavicle, long-bone
  - any paralysis
- failed instrumental delivery, proceeding to caesarean section
- low cord pH
- major congenital abnormalities first detected at delivery
- any event considered to be serious, regardless of outcome.

Why do we need clinical incident analysis?

Obstetrics accounts for a significant fraction of all claims and the largest proportion of damages paid in clinical negligence litigation.

By continual review of clinical incidents, we will be able to improve patient care and reduce risks to patients as follows:

- Near-misses are an important source of information to prevent such accidents happening again.
- Identification of common themes can help to predict and prevent future incidents.
- Early warning signs can be picked up.

We can promote a culture of learning and enquiry, and help all members of the multidisciplinary team to reflect on their practice and make changes as necessary. The principle is not to blame or shame, but to promote active learning and improve the quality of care.

Clinical incidents are commonly due to inadequacies in the system rather than the fault of an individual. Analysis of incidents will be used to determine how the system can be improved, and not to punish the individual. The analysis will be used to identify unexpected events and those with poor outcomes that may need further investigation. Once patterns emerge, we can focus on prevention and education. Information could alert line managers to possible weaknesses in systems of work.

Clinical incident analysis will provide an archive of facts for possible use in medico-legal cases.

Reporting clinical incidents

Incidents should be reported using the Trust's incident-reporting form and in line with the Trust's risk management strategy.

During the weekly intrapartum care meeting, practitioners are encouraged to present unusual cases or those with a suboptimal outcome. The practitioner will complete and submit the 'Critical Case Analysis' form to the Risk Management Midwife.

Analysis of clinical incidents

In addition to use of the incident reporting system, the unit will identify clinical incidents through its computer database. Using the trigger list, the maternity information system manager will generate a list of cases for review each month.

The Risk Management Midwife will then distribute cases to experienced midwives and doctors for peer review. Experienced practitioners are encouraged to involve junior colleagues in the review process.

After reviewing the case(s), the midwife or doctor completes the 'Critical Case Analysis' form, and returns it to the Risk Management Midwife within 28 days. The reviewer indicates on the form whether they believe that the case should go for second review by a consultant obstetrician and/or a supervisor of midwives, as appropriate. The reviewer also indicates on the form whether the case is suitable for presentation in the multidisciplinary audit meeting.

The Risk Management Midwife collates and reviews the completed forms. These forms may be disclosed in legal proceedings. They should be stored in line with the local policy. In the vast majority of cases, clinical care has been good and no further action is required. Where further action is required, follow the Trust's risk management policy.

If there are unresolved issues, the case is referred to a consultant obstetrician or a supervisor of midwives for second review. Some incidents will require in-depth investigation ('root cause analysis'); this will be arranged by the Risk Management Midwife. The directorate's Risk Management Committee, in concert with directorate management, is responsible for implementing any recommendations arising from the reporting and investigation of clinical incidents.

The Risk Management Midwife will inform the directorate audit lead if a particular case or a trend has identified the need for an audit of practice.

Confidentiality

Practitioners are expected to respect the confidentiality of their colleagues when undertaking a review. Information will be handled at all times in a way that protects patients' confidentiality, and in keeping with the Data Protection Act. Anonymous reporting is preferable to concealment. Incidents or near-misses may be reported anonymously or (preferably) confidentially to the ward manager, the consultant or the Risk Management Midwife.

Transfer of care between professionals

Background

This guidance stems from recommendations by various bodies concerned with quality of care:

- CNST standards call for clear arrangements concerning which professional is responsible for the patient's care at all times.
- The Confidential Enquiries into Stillbirths and Deaths in Infancy (CESDI) emphasizes the importance of adequate arrangements for transfer of patients between units.
- The Royal Colleges, in the document *Towards Safer Childbirth*, state that explicit lines of communication between professionals are crucial to optimization of birth outcomes.

Handover by medical staff on labour ward

There should be a personal handover on the ward at 0830, 1300 and 1700 on weekdays, and at 0900 at weekends. The handover takes priority over other, non-emergency clinical duties.

It is unacceptable to leave the bleep at the ward station or reception.

Transfer of emergencies from primary care

Emergency transfers to the labour ward can be made at any time by the GP or community midwife after discussion with the medical or midwifery staff. The team leader/coordinator must be informed. Some referrals will be more appropriate to the antenatal day assessment unit or the early pregnancy assessment unit and should be directed accordingly.

Transfer between hospitals with the fetus *in utero*

- ☐ All transfers in or out must be with the prior approval of the consultant obstetrician.
- ☐ If there is a good chance that the baby will need to be delivered in the next 48 hours, then availability of a cot in the neonatal unit of the receiving hospital must be confirmed before transfer.
- ☐ Where indicated, prophylactic steroids should be given before transfer in or out.
- ☐ Where indicated, a tocolytic should be given before transfer in or out.

☐ Appropriate personnel should accompany the woman. The coordinating midwife and the consultant obstetrician will determine the appropriate personnel for each case.

☐ Do not transfer (or accept a transfer) if any of the following applies:
- uncontrolled vaginal bleeding
- cervix >4 cm dilated
- three or more uterine contractions in 10 minutes.

☐ A letter and a copy (not the original) of the notes should accompany the woman.

☐ Results of relevant investigations should be recorded in the notes or telephoned through to the receiving hospital as soon as available.

Transfer of care between consultants

When a patient is referred to a special or subspecialty clinic, there should be a referral letter indicating whether this is an outright transfer or a request for opinion only.

For emergency admission of unbooked patients, the woman is under the consultant on call at the time of admission, unless she has an unfinished clinical episode under another consultant, in which case she remains under that consultant's care. A clinical episode, in this context, finishes when a discharge letter has been written.

Transfer back to the community or GP care

Follow-up plans/arrangements should always be specified in the case notes (hospital and hand-held) and in discharge letters. If no follow-up appointment has been arranged, then this should be stated in a discharge letter.

Following a stillbirth, miscarriage or termination for fetal anomaly, the GP, community midwife and health visitor must be informed immediately (see also pp. 207–208).

Where it has been arranged for a patient to be followed up by the community midwife, this should be documented in the case notes and in the diary kept on the unit.

Transfer to ITU and HDU

Who transfers?

A patient may be transferred to ITU or surgical HDU at the request of the consultant obstetrician/gynaecologist, consultant anaesthetist or anaesthetic registrar. All transfers to ITU must be discussed first with the consultant anaesthetist in charge.

Who is in charge while the patient is in ITU or HDU?

The patient in ITU is primarily under the care of the consultant anaesthetist, but the consultant obstetrician/gynaecologist remains responsible for the obstetric/gynaecological care. Any woman admitted into ITU must be seen daily by the obstetric team.

The consultant obstetrician/gynaecologist is primarily responsible for the care of his or her patient transferred to the HDU.

Reviewing what happened

It is often helpful if the newly delivered mother has an opportunity to discuss her experience with a professional who was involved in her care. Events are reviewed and, where necessary, issues are clarified.

The review provides the opportunity for the mother to:

- ask questions
- express her feelings, eg pleasure, gratitude, fear, anger, confusion, other emotions
- understand the reasons for unmet expectations
- be reassured of her success and her achievement
- plan for future pregnancies.

The review should be held at a mutually convenient time before discharge. The format of the review is not prescriptive. It should be a listening and sharing activity, not a counselling activity.

A summary of the following should be recorded in the postnatal records:

- [ ] Date and time of meeting.
- [ ] Matters discussed.
- [ ] Questions asked.
- [ ] Unresolved issues, if any.
- [ ] Further action required.

Where difficulties are experienced, support and advice should be sought from a ward manager, supervisor or consultant.

Some women may prefer to speak with a midwife or obstetrician not involved in the delivery.

If a complaint is imminent, then the Trust's complaint policy should be followed.

Further reading

Communication

NHS Litigation Authority. Criteria 3.14 and 3.15. In: *Clinical Negligence Scheme for Trusts Clinical Risk Management Standards for Maternity Services*. London: NHS Litigation Authority, 2002.

Royal College of Obstetricians and Gynaecologists. *Clinical Standards. Advice on Planning the Service in Obstetrics and Gynaecology*. London: RCOG Press, 2002.

Royal College of Obstetricians and Gynaecologists and Royal College of Midwives. *Towards Safer Childbirth. Minimum Standards for the Organisation of Labour Wards. Report of a Joint Working Party*. London: RCOG Press, 1999.

Documentation

Cowan J. Clinical governance and clinical documentation: still a long way to go? *Clin Perform Qual Health Care* 2000; **8**: 179–82.

NHS Litigation Authority. Standard 6. In: *Clinical Negligence Scheme for Trusts Clinical Risk Management Standards for Maternity Services*. London: NHS Litigation Authority, 2002.

UK Central Council for Nursing, Midwifery and Health Visiting. *Guidelines for Records and Record Keeping*. London: UK Central Council for Nursing, Midwifery and Health Visiting, 1998.

UK Central Council for Nursing, Midwifery and Health Visiting. Rule 42. In: *Midwives Rules and Code of Practice*. London: UK Central Council for Nursing, Midwifery and Health Visiting, 1998.

Clinical incident reporting

Department of Health. *An Organisation with a Memory. Report of an Expert Group on Learning from Adverse Events in the NHS*. London: The Stationary Office, 2000.

NHS Litigation Authority. *Clinical Negligence Scheme for Trusts Clinical Risk Management Standards for Maternity Services*, version 01. London: NHS Litigation Authority, 2000.

Section 2: Normal and low-risk labour

'To view [labour] as a temporary aberration from normal, or as a temporary illness, obscures some of the positive developmental processes that are possible. That is not to overlook the abnormal developments which may take place during labour and require urgent intervention'

– Prince J, Adams ME. *Minds, Mothers and Midwives – The Psychology of Childbirth*. London: Churchill Livingstone 1978, p. 118

Vaginal examination

Before vaginal examination:

☐ A history should be taken.
☐ Ultrasound scan results should be noted.
☐ Consent must be obtained.
☐ Abdominal examination and auscultation should be performed.

The following details should be recorded:

☐ Date and time.
☐ Findings on abdominal examination
☐ Indication for vaginal examination.
☐ Relevant information on condition of external genitalia and vagina.
☐ Cervical effacement.
☐ Cervical dilatation.
☐ Presentation
   – level of presenting part in relation to ischial spines
   – application to cervix
   – caput
   – moulding
      +   skull bones apposed
      ++   reducible overlap of bones
      +++ irreducible overlap of bones.
☐ Membranes
   – intact or absent
   – colour and volume of amniotic fluid.
☐ Fetal heart auscultation following procedure.
☐ Findings explained to mother.
☐ Signature and print name.

Intravenous cannulation

Intravenous cannulation is required for patients with:

- high-risk pregnancy
- previous postpartum haemorrhage
- grandmultiparity (fifth and subsequent labours)
- anaemia ([Hb] <10 g/dl)
- previous caesarean section (undergoing a trial of vaginal delivery)
- meconium-stained amniotic fluid.

10 ml of blood for group-and-save serum and FBC to be sent to the laboratory.

All group-and-save serum samples must be signed by two professionals.

The cannula should be flushed using either 5 ml normal saline or 5 ml Hepsal.

Syntocinon infusion may be commenced as per patient group direction when:

- induction of labour has been agreed previously by obstetrician
- there is slow progress and the obstetrician on call has confirmed that labour should be augmented.

All indications, discussions and agreement should be documented.

In the event of PPH occurring, an infusion of 500 ml Hartmann's solution and 40 units Syntocinon may be commenced whilst awaiting medical assistance.

No intravenous fluids other than those indicated on the patient group direction should be given without being prescribed by a doctor.

Management of normal labour

Normal labour will be managed by the midwifery staff.

Criteria for normal labour

Normal labour is defined by the presence of all of the following criteria:

- [ ] Uncomplicated pregnancy (most will have been booked for midwifery-led care).
- [ ] Spontaneous onset of labour at 37–40 weeks' gestation.
- [ ] Minimum rate of cervical dilation 1 cm/hour from diagnosis of established labour.
- [ ] First referral to labour ward.
- [ ] Single fetus with engaged head.
- [ ] Clear amniotic fluid.
- [ ] Normal maternal observations.
- [ ] No intrapartum bleeding.
- [ ] No maternal or fetal distress.
- [ ] Normal delivery within one hour of good expulsive effort.
- [ ] Intact perineum, first- or second-degree tear or episiotomy.
- [ ] Third stage lasts for less than 20 minutes following active management.
- [ ] Immediate postpartum blood loss <500 ml.

The SHO or registrar should be called to see any woman falling outside these criteria.

Prelabour rupture of membranes at term (37–42 weeks)

A woman with suspected spontaneous rupture of membranes and no associated contractions or vaginal bleeding may be assessed (CTG, sterile speculum examination) on the antenatal ward or day unit.

If the woman is bleeding or has uterine contractions, then she should be admitted to the delivery suite.

An experienced midwife may perform a speculum examination and obtain a vaginal swab provided the following criteria are met:

- normal uneventful pregnancy at 37–40 weeks
- normal fetal heart rate
- no vaginal bleeding
- consent obtained.

The mother may be observed on the antenatal ward if prelabour rupture of membranes (PROM) is confirmed and the following criteria are met:

- no meconium-stained amniotic fluid
- cephalic presentation, well-applied to the cervix
- normal maternal observations
- <24 hours have elapsed since rupture of membranes
- vaginal swab has been taken.

If any of these criteria does not apply, then the obstetrician on call should be informed.

Where PROM is excluded, the discharge protocol should be followed.

Further management

Women with confirmed PROM should be offered a choice of expectant management (not exceeding 72 hours) or immediate induction of labour.

The benefits and risks of expectant management versus immediate induction of labour should be discussed, and the agreed plan should be documented.

Expectant management

Await spontaneous onset of labour. If labour does not ensue, induce after 12–72 hours (as agreed with the woman).

Induction protocol (see p. 82 for details):

- *Bishop score <5:* prostaglandin 1 mg (or 2 mg if nulliparous). Reassess six hours later if not in labour.
- *Bishop score ≥5:* Syntocinon infusion.

When 18 hours have elapsed since rupture of membranes, antibiotics should be given (see p. 177).

Active management

Induce with prostaglandin or Syntocinon, as above. See p. 82 for protocol for induction of labour.

(An alternative, but unlicensed, option is active management with oral misoprostol 50 µg, repeated every four hours if required, to a maximum of five doses. In the Aberdeen study, nine out of 10 women on this regime were in labour within 24 hours. Uterine rupture following induction of labour with misoprostol has been reported, and the dose stated above should not be exceeded.)

Management of first stage of labour

Diagnosis

It is important to get the diagnosis of labour right, as this is the fundamental decision on which all subsequent management is based. Diagnosis is based on painful, regular contractions along with one or more of the following:

- 'show'
- spontaneous rupture of membranes
- cervical effacement and dilatation on vaginal examination >2 cm (primipara) or >3 cm (multipara).

Monitoring progress of labour

If the woman is in established labour, then her progress and wellbeing should be assessed and managed by her named midwife, who will be aware at all times of the patient's wishes.

Commence partogram and record all maternal and fetal observations. Pulse rate should be recorded every half-hour. Temperature should be recorded every four hours if apyrexial, but every hour if pyrexial. Blood pressure should be recorded every half-hour if the woman is hypertensive or having epidural analgesia; in other cases, blood pressure should be recorded every two hours.

Descent of the presenting part should be assessed abdominally (fifths palpable, see Glossary, p. 235) and vaginally (centimetres above or below the ischial spines). Do not rely on vaginal examination only, as caput and moulding may give a false impression of lower descent.

Repeat vaginal examinations at three-hourly intervals unless there is a reason to examine at shorter intervals.

Birth plans

Birth plans should be respected and supported as much as possible.

If any change in the birth plan becomes necessary, this should be discussed with the mother and a record made. Engaging the mother in this way enhances her birth experience.

Support person

The continuous presence of a midwife or other support person reduces the likelihood of operative delivery or low Apgar score. It is also associated with a shorter duration of labour and reduced requirement for analgesia.

A link worker should be present if needed or requested.

Positioning

The adoption of the upright position during labour will facilitate efficient uterine contractions, shorten the latent phase and reduce the need for analgesia. The woman should be encouraged to move around and adopt whatever position she finds most comfortable during labour.

Nutrition

The woman in labour needs energy and should not be starved unless she is likely to require a general anaesthetic. If she is in normal labour, the mother may have a high-carbohydrate/low-fat diet if she wishes.

Fluids may be taken freely in normal labour. When surgery is anticipated, non-particulate, non-fizzy drinks may be taken up to two hours before an operation.

Antacids

Antacid prophylaxis should be given selectively in labour to women considered to be at high risk for operative intervention.

Any woman requiring IV cannulation will usually fall into the high-risk group. Indications include previous CS, multiple pregnancy, abnormal lie or presentation, preterm labour, diabetes, APH, and non-reassuring CTG.

Dose: ranitidine 150 mg orally every six hours until completion of the third stage. Women who are vomiting, who have had opioid analgesia, or who are otherwise unable to take oral medication should be given ranitidine 50 mg IM six-hourly.

Women not in labour but undergoing a 'crash' CS should have IV ranitidine 50 mg in 20 ml normal saline over 2 minutes and IV metoclopramide 10 mg. See also p. 71.

Pain relief

The woman should be informed of the various methods of pain relief that are available. The analgesia requested should be administered and documented as per patient group direction. For epidural analgesia, see p. 36.

Anti-infective filters or fully disposable breathing systems should be used with Entonox apparatus.

Fetal monitoring

A risk assessment is done on admission to the delivery suite.

For low-risk women, the fetal heart may be auscultated intermittently using a fetal stethoscope (Pinard) or Doppler (Sonicaid). Auscultate for 60 seconds, beginning immediately after the end of a contraction, every 15 minutes in the first stage of labour and every 5 minutes in the second stage. See pp. 4–5 for a list of some conditions that exclude women from this group.

For at-risk women, a CTG is mandatory on admission. Continuous electronic monitoring is required in the following situations:

- epidural sited
- Syntocinon infusion in progress
- fresh meconium-stained amniotic fluid
- high-risk pregnancy (maternal or fetal problems)
- maternal request
- intermittent auscultation reveals decelerations
- baseline <110 or >160 beats/min.

☐ Before commencing CTG or intermittent auscultation, palpate the maternal pulse simultaneously with auscultation to differentiate between maternal and fetal heart rates.
☐ Check that the date and time clocks on the monitor are set correctly.
☐ Ensure that the paper speed is set to 1 cm/min.
☐ Label the paper with the woman's identifying details.
☐ If a good trace cannot be obtained using an abdominal transducer, then use a scalp electrode. If the signal is still poor, then the presence of fetal heart pulsation should be confirmed by an ultrasound scan.

Fetal scalp electrodes are contraindicated in:

- women with HIV or hepatitis virus
- fetal bleeding disorder (eg haemophilia).

Suspicious or abnormal trace

If any fetal heart rate abnormality is identified, then monitoring should be continuous and, where necessary, a fetal scalp electrode applied. The team leader should be informed; if they are not happy, then the registrar on call should be asked to review.

Any midwife or doctor reviewing a trace should document on both the trace and the case notes, stating their findings and plan.

When describing and acting on a CTG, the following features should be documented:

☐ Frequency and strength of uterine contractions.
☐ Baseline fetal heart rate.
☐ Variability.
☐ Presence or absence of accelerations.
☐ Presence or absence of decelerations.
☐ Overall assessment and plan, taking into account any background risk.

Classification of cardiotocograph (see Table 1)

■ *Normal:* all four features of the cardiograph are normal.
■ *Suspicious:* one feature is non-reassuring.
■ *Pathological:* two features are non-reassuring, or there is at least one abnormal feature.

Table 1 *Classification of cardiotocograph*

Classification	Baseline (beats/min)	Variability	Deceleration	Acceleration
Reassuring	110–160	≥5	None	Present
Non-reassuring	100–109, 161–180	<5 for 40–90 min	Early deceleration Variable deceleration Deceleration for ≤3 min	
Abnormal	<100, >180 Sinusoidal pattern for ≥10 min	<5 for ≥90 min	Late deceleration Atypical variable deceleration Prolonged deceleration for >3 min	

Management of suspicious or pathological cardiotocograph

☐ Adopt left lateral position.
☐ Inform registrar.
☐ Exclude hypotension; give crystalloid infusion if appropriate.
☐ Exclude hypercontractility; stop Syntocinon infusion.
☐ Check maternal pulse and temperature.
☐ Exclude cord prolapse (vaginal examination).
☐ If trace is pathological or persistently suspicious, then fetal blood sampling is indicated (see p. 30).

Do not give oxygen to the mother, as it may be harmful to the hypoxic baby

Management of fetal tachycardia

Ask the following questions:

- Is there an obvious explanation?
- How severe is the tachycardia?
- Are there other complications (decelerations, loss of variability) on the CTG?
- Is delivery imminent?

Take the following action:

- ☐ Check maternal pulse and temperature.
- ☐ Correct dehydration.
- ☐ If fetal heart rate is 160–180 beats/min and trace is uncomplicated, no intervention is required
- ☐ If persistent and >180 beats/min, do fetal blood sampling. If FBS not feasible, discuss with consultant and proceed to CS.

Note: In cases of fetal sepsis there could be tachycardia with normal fetal scalp blood pH. Bear this in mind where there has been prolonged rupture of fetal membranes.

Management of fetal bradycardia

Assess the following:

- depth of bradycardia
- duration of bradycardia
- signs of recovery (rapid or slow?)
- variability
- nature of the trace prior to bradycardia
- if in second stage, is delivery imminent?

Take the following action:

- ☐ Left lateral tilt.
- ☐ Turn off Syntocinon infusion.
- ☐ Check and record maternal pulse.
- ☐ Check blood pressure.
- ☐ If hypotensive or has just had epidural, give rapid infusion of IV fluid. (Note: following epidural, a drop in fetal heart rate may occur even with a normal blood pressure.)
- ☐ Vaginal examination to exclude cord prolapse and to assess cervix and descent.
- ☐ If there is vaginal bleeding, then consider possibility of placental abruption or uterine rupture.
- ☐ If not recovering by six minutes, prepare for operative delivery (CS or instrumental).

Scalp pH should not be performed for prolonged bradycardia.

If there is bradycardia lasting up to 10 minutes, then proceed straight to CS (or instrumental delivery if feasible).

The schedule is as follows:

- *1–5 minutes:* call for help. Review as outlined above.
- *6 minutes:* expect recovery towards baseline. If not recovering, prepare for operative delivery.
- *9 minutes:* if no recovery, transfer to theatre (or effect instrumental delivery if feasible).
- *15 minutes:* baby delivered.

Reduced variability (2–5 beats/min)

- May reflect fetal sleep.
- Has the mother had narcotic drug or sedation?
- If it lasts longer than 40 minutes, do FBS (or discuss with consultant if FBS not feasible).

Absent variability (<2 beats/min) calls for immediate intervention.

Note: When interpreting a complicated CTG, pay particular attention to the variability.

A more accurate picture of variability is obtained from a scalp electrode than from an abdominal transducer. The latter tends to overestimate variability.

Late deceleration

Take the following action:

☐ Left lateral tilt.
☐ Turn off Syntocinon infusion.
☐ Check blood pressure.
☐ Vaginal examination to exclude cord prolapse and to assess cervix and descent.
☐ If cervix ≥3 cm dilated, do FBS. If cervix <3 cm dilated, proceed to CS.

Decelerations in the second stage of labour may be innocent or indicative of hypoxia. Assess the following: – nature of trace in the first stage of labour
– depth, duration and recovery of decelerations
– variability

If these give cause for concern, then operative delivery is indicated (see also 'Contraindications to fetal blood sampling', p. 30).

Fetal scalp blood sampling

If the CTG is suggestive of fetal distress, then fetal scalp blood sampling (FBS) should always be undertaken before proceeding to CS, unless it is technically not possible to do so.

☐ Explain the procedure to the patient and obtain consent.
☐ Cervix must be at least 3 cm dilated and the presenting part should be no more than 2 cm above plane of ischial spines.
☐ Left lateral position. Alternatively, lithotomy position with wedge.
☐ At least two samples should be taken on each occasion. After obtaining sample, ensure haemostasis by applying pressure with a swab on the stab site.
☐ Inform patient of result and plan.

Contraindications to fetal blood sampling

The following are contraindications to fetal blood sampling:

- prolonged (>10 minutes) fetal bradycardia
- pathological CTG associated with antepartum haemorrhage, suspected chorioamnionitis, or possible rupture of uterine scar
- pregnancy <34 weeks
- full cervical dilatation and presenting part below spines (*deliver the baby!*)
- HIV-positive or hepatitis B-positive/C-positive mother.

Interpretation of pH result

Normal values:

- pH >7.25
- pO_2 >2.6 kPa (>20 mmHg) (note: pO_2 is not of value in assessing risk to the baby)
- pCO_2 <8 kPa (<50 mmHg)
- base excess >8 mEq/l.

Results should be interpreted in the context of the clinical features, rate of progress in labour, and the previous pH reading:

- *≥7.25:* normal; may need repeating if CTG abnormality persists
- *≤7.20:* acidosis; delivery indicated
- *7.21–7.24:* repeat within 30 minutes, or consider delivery if rapid fall since last sample.

If two neat samples were obtained, management should be based on the lower pH. If no good sample was obtained, FBS should be repeated – do not derive false reassurance from an inadequate sample.

Documentation

☐ Verbal consent.
☐ pH meter printout, labelled and dated, should be secured with sticky tape in the case notes.
☐ Plan of management following blood sampling.

Fetal blood sampling at full cervical dilatation

If the cervix is fully dilated and the presenting part is below the plane of the ischial spines, then the woman should be offered instrumental delivery.

If the presenting part is still high, FBS may be performed. A normal result allows time for descent of the presenting part, thus allowing a normal delivery or increasing the chances of a successful instrumental delivery.

If FBS has been performed, then cord-blood sampling must be performed at delivery.

Augmentation of labour

If labour is slow, consider the following possible causes:

- prolonged latent phase of labour (safe to augment)
- inefficient uterine activity (generally safe to augment)
- obstructed labour (dangerous to augment).

Artificial rupture of membranes

'The older doctrine of the sanctity of the membranes was more or less built in with the bricks in my obstetrical philosophy. No labour is so pleasing and satisfactory to mother and child as when intact membranes are maintained right up to full dilatation at which point a gush of clear, clean liquor amnii flushes out the genital tract, followed, not so many minutes later, by the delivery of a clean, healthy, screaming baby. This is Nature at her best and I never cease to marvel at such normality'. – Donald I. *Practical Obstetric Problems*, 5th edn. London: Lloyd-Luke, 1979, p. 566.

Artificial rupture of membranes (ARM) should not be performed routinely, but it may be used to accelerate labour if progress is slow (<1 cm/hour).

The rate of progress must be considered in the context of the mother's circumstances. A rate of 1 cm/hour in a woman who is having strong uterine contractions and who is in severe distress is more worrying than a rate of 0.5 cm/hour in a woman who is comfortable and mobile.

The midwife may rupture the membranes artificially (for induction or augmentation of labour) if the following criteria are met and the mother consents:

☐ Head is engaged.
☐ Vertex is presenting.
☐ Cord presentation has been excluded.

Contraindications to ARM are:

- abnormal lie
- cord presentation
- placenta praevia.

After ARM, check for cord prolapse and meconium staining of amniotic fluid. Document the fetal heart rate.

Augmentation with Syntocinon

Syntocinon may be prescribed to accelerate labour provided that the following conditions are met:

☐ Presentation is cephalic.
☐ Membranes have ruptured.
☐ Amniotic fluid is clear.

Syntocinon infusion should not be started until six hours have elapsed since administration of prostaglandin.

Syntocinon should not be used in secondary arrest (after 5 cm dilatation) until obstructed labour has been excluded by vaginal examination. Particular care should be taken in multiparous women.

The use of Syntocinon in the following circumstances requires the explicit approval of the consultant:

- multiple pregnancy
- malpresentation
- previous caesarean section or other uterine scar
- grandmultiparity.

If augmentation of labour is indicated, then the midwife, per patient group direction, may commence an intravenous infusion of Syntocinon:

- if maternal and fetal wellbeing are normal
- following discussion with obstetrician on call
- with documentation in labour records.

Syntocinon infusion

Mix 10 units of Syntocinon in 500 ml Hartmann's solution. Commence infusion at 2 milliunits/min (ie 6 ml/hour). Increase every 30 minutes until strong, regular uterine contractions – three in 10 minutes – are obtained.

A syringe driver or infusion pump must be used.

Do not exceed 32 milliunits/min (ie 96 ml/hour); see Table 2.

Do not infuse through the same line as blood, plasma or insulin.

The syringe must be labelled, with the dose of drug and signatures of responsible staff on the label.

All women for whom labour is being augmented with Syntocinon should have continuous electronic fetal monitoring.

Table 2 *Regimen for Syntocinon infusion*

Time after starting (min)	Rate (milliunits/min)	Rate (ml/h)
0	2	6
30	4	12
60	8	24
90	12	36
120	16	48
150	20	60
180	24	72
210	28	84
240	32	96

Second stage of labour

Syntocinon infusion may be given to augment uterine contractions in the second stage of labour, providing that obstructed labour has been excluded by abdominal and vaginal examination.

Mix 10 units of Syntocinon in 500 ml Hartmann's solution. Commence infusion at 2 milliunits/min (ie 6 ml/hour). Increase every 15 minutes until strong, regular uterine contractions – three in 10 minutes – are obtained.

Uterine hyperstimulation

Definition:

- more than five contractions per 10 minutes for at least 20 minutes or each uterine contraction lasting at least 2 minutes
- suspicious or pathological CTG.

Management:

☐ Discontinue Syntocinon infusion.
☐ Lie on left side.
☐ Rapid infusion of 1000 ml normal saline.
☐ In extreme cases, consider tocolysis with terbutaline 0.25 mg SC.
☐ It may be necessary to deliver the baby – is the CTG back to normal?

Cord-blood sampling

Blood should be obtained for acid–base status from an isolated segment of umbilical cord following delivery of any potentially acidotic fetus, including:

- abnormal intrapartum CTG
- cases where fetal scalp blood has been sampled
- instrumental vaginal delivery
- preterm delivery
- breech vaginal delivery
- intrauterine growth restriction
- placental abruption
- cord prolapse
- baby born with low Apgar score
- fetal abnormality.

A quality control check must be made on the analyser as directed by the manufacturer (see handbook accompanying machine).

A 10 cm segment of cord is clamped immediately after delivery of the baby.

Samples of cord artery and vein are obtained with pre-heparinized syringes.

The segment of cord (or sample in pre-heparinized syringe) may be left at room temperature for up to 30 minutes, or in ice for up to one hour, before analysis.

Inform the duty paediatrician if arterial pH is <7.05 or if venous pH is <7.20.

 Beware – with some analysers, the quality control printout could be mistaken for the actual specimen result

Epidural analgesia in labour

Epidural analgesia in labour requires a resident anaesthetist and continuous care and monitoring of the mother and fetus by a suitably trained midwife. If either is unavailable, then epidural analgesia should not be instituted. Patient information about epidurals and other forms of pain relief is available in the antenatal clinic and on the delivery unit. Various translations are available.

Indications

- maternal request
- occipitoposterior position
- induced/accelerated labour
- prolonged labour
- multiple pregnancy
- breech presentation
- pre-eclampsia (see below)
- premature birth/high-risk fetus
- maternal medical problems, eg diabetes, asthma, certain cardiac problems.

Contraindications

- maternal refusal
- coagulopathy (see below)
- shock/uncorrected hypovolaemia
- inadequate staffing
- septicaemia
- local infection
- raised intracranial pressure
- allergy to amide local anaesthetics (rare).

Coagulopathy

The risks and benefits of epidural analgesia/anaesthesia need to be assessed in each case. It is not possible to lay down absolute criteria. Regional block would usually be given if the platelet count is above 100×10^9/l, but epidural analgesia may be withheld if the count is higher than this but falling rapidly. A coagulation profile must be done if the platelet count is <100, and a senior anaesthetist must be involved.

A platelet count should be done in pre-eclampsia and where there has previously been a low count.

In addition, PT, APTT and FDPs should be checked in the following cases:

- severe pre-eclampsia (including HELLP)
- intrauterine death
- placental abruption.

Therapeutic/prophylactic anticoagulation

See also pp. 144, 149.

Some women will have had low-molecular-weight heparin (LMWH, usually daltepatin [Fragmin]) for prophylaxis or treatment of thrombosis. This is not an absolute contraindication to regional block.

Peak anti-Xa activity (see Glossary, p. 235) is reached about three hours after a subcutaneous injection of LMWH, but 50% of peak levels are still present at 12 hours. Spinal/epidural should be inserted at least 12 hours after a prophylactic dose and 24 hours after a therapeutic dose. Patients on any anticoagulant should have PT and APTT checked before placing an epidural/spinal, but note that these are unlikely to be affected by LMWH.

Setting up

Exact equipment requirements vary between anaesthetists. The following are usually required:

☐ IV cannula (minimum 16G, ie grey Venflon) with 1000 ml bag of Hartmann's solution connected via a blood-giving set.
☐ Epidural trolley, fully stocked (stock list is on the trolley).
☐ Resuscitation equipment, including oxygen and suction.
☐ Patient's records and an epidural chart.
☐ Blood pressure and fetal heart monitoring equipment.
☐ Tilting bed.
☐ Wedge.

The anaesthetist will want to know:

- parity
- previous epidural?
- stage and progress of labour
- other analgesia used
- significant obstetric and medical problems
- maternal blood pressure and vaginal examination findings.

The procedure

☐ Procedure explained by the anaesthetist; verbal consent obtained and documented.
☐ Ask the woman to empty her bladder.
☐ Preload of IV fluid may be given. The drip must be able to flow freely if needed.

☐ Woman either on her side or sitting on the side of the bed and leaning over a table.
☐ Appropriate area of the back (L2–3 or L3–4) cleaned with chlorhexidine spray.
☐ The midwife should support the mother during the procedure, particularly with regard to maintaining good position.
☐ After catheter insertion, a test dose of local anaesthetic is given to exclude placement in the cerebrospinal fluid or a vein.
☐ Blood pressure and pulse rate should be checked every five minutes for a further 20 minutes, during which time the mother should not be left unattended.

Method of administration:

When the epidural catheter has been inserted, continuous analgesia can be administered by one of the following means:

- continuous infusion
- intermittent boluses (top-ups)
- patient-controlled epidural analgesia
- combined spinal epidural.

Epidural infusion

Continuous infusion reduces, but does not eliminate, the need for bolus injections. Often at least one top-up is required. There are two reasons for this:

- Epidural drug requirements tend to increase as labour progresses.
- Infusion rates sufficient to eliminate the need for top-ups often cause excessive blocks and are therefore best avoided.

The anaesthetist will prescribe the anaesthetic agent (eg 0.2% ropivacaine or 0.25% bupivacaine), and the infusion rate. When indicated, the infusion rate should be adjusted as outlined in Table 3.

The following observations are required hourly:

☐ Volume infused.
☐ Infusion rate.
☐ Presence or absence of excessive motor block (inability to bend both knees).
☐ Block height (test for cold sensation or pinch in the epigastrium; sensation should be normal here).

Table 3 *Adjustments to infusion rate when there is a problem*

Finding	Action
Mother in pain	Administer top-up (see next page) and increase rate by 2 ml/h
Epigastric cold/pinch	Reduce rate by 2 ml/h
Sensation abnormal	Recheck in 30 min
Excessive motor block	Reduce rate by 2 ml/h
	Recheck in 30 min

Inform anaesthetist if:

■ pain does not respond to a top-up after 20 minutes
■ abnormal epigastric sensation persists 30 minutes after reducing infusion rate
■ excessive motor block persists 30 minutes after reducing infusion rate.

Epidural top-up

A trained midwife may give top-ups of anaesthetic in doses prescribed by the anaesthetist. The anaesthetist must be available within 5 minutes if there are problems. Typical doses are 10–15 ml 0.125% bupivacaine or 15 ml of 0.1% bupivacaine with 2 mg/ml fentanyl, given every hour.

Protocol for top-ups

☐ A top-up is indicated if the mother is in pain and feels that her analgesia is inadequate.
☐ Check epidural prescription (*do not rely on oral instructions*).
☐ Check maternal pulse and blood pressure, motor block and block height. Contact anaesthetist if any adverse findings.
☐ Check bladder fullness and empty as necessary.
☐ Draw up prescribed dose of anaesthetic agent. *This must be checked with a second midwife.*
☐ Do not administer epidural drugs during a contraction.
☐ The mother should be in sitting or full lateral position.
☐ Administer drug in a divided dose.
☐ Initial fraction given *slowly*. Over the next five minutes, observe/ask about sudden increase in motor block, dizziness, tingling in the face and tinnitus
☐ At five minutes, check maternal pulse and blood pressure. *Note: upper arm will under-read blood pressure if patient is in lateral position.* If dizziness, tingling or other symptom is observed or if systolic blood pressure falls below 90 mmHg (or by more than 30 mmHg), then omit the remaining fraction and call the anaesthetist. Otherwise, administer the remaining dose and continue observing for these symptoms or hypotension.
☐ Check blood pressure every five minutes for a further 20 minutes. The mother must not be left unattended during this time

> **!** If the top-up is ineffective after 20 minutes, call the anaesthetist.

If hypotension occurs at any stage, treat as outlined under 'Hypotension' on pp. 40–41 and call the anaesthetist.

General care of the woman with an epidural

The woman should be looked after by a dedicated and suitably trained midwife. The anaesthetist remains responsible for the regional block and should attend regularly, not just when called by the midwife.

If the midwife has any concerns about the epidural (see complications below) the anaesthetist should be contacted.

The woman should never be supine. If the woman is on her back, then a wedge must be under the right buttock at all times, even during vaginal examination. At other times, the sitting position is preferred. If the woman wishes to lie down, then the full lateral position is acceptable.

☐ Hourly position changes (to avoid pressure-related problems) recorded on the appropriate chart and continued until the epidural has worn off completely.
☐ Maternal blood pressure checked every 30 minutes.
☐ Continuous fetal heart monitoring (note: CTG abnormalities may occur up to 1 hour after epidural).
☐ Temperature checked every four hours.
☐ Encourage bladder emptying every two hours and before top-ups. Regular palpation to detect urinary retention. Record urine output
☐ Vaginal examination as indicated (with wedge in place).

In the second stage of labour:

- Breakthrough pain may occur. A top-up should be offered. This should be given in the sitting position to block the sacral root.
- The epidural infusion should not be stopped. If the woman is totally unaware of her contractions (not common in practice), then she should be encouraged to push when contractions are palpated. The prescribed infusion rate may be reduced by 2 ml/hour in these circumstances.
- A second-stage duration of two hours is acceptable if maternal and fetal conditions allow.
- Perineal infiltration may still be required before episiotomy.

Complications
Inadequate analgesia

- May occur at some stage in up to 20% of epidurals.
- Give a top-up as detailed above and call the anaesthetist if ineffective after 20 minutes.

Hypotension

Prevention:

- Make appropriate checks before giving a bolus.

- Avoid the supine position at all times.
- Correct pre-existing hypovolaemia.

If systolic blood pressure falls below 90 mmHg (on lower arm if in the lateral position):

☐ Turn to full lateral position. If this is ineffective, then:
☐ Fully open the drip and give 500 ml compound sodium lactate (Hartmann's solution).
☐ Give oxygen by facemask (minimum 10 litres flow with wall oxygen).
☐ Call the anaesthetist.
☐ Have ready a box of ephedrine, water for dilution and a 10-ml syringe.

Dural tap

- Occurs when the epidural needle or catheter accidentally penetrates the dura, usually resulting in a leak of cerebrospinal fluid.
- Immediate management varies between cases. The anaesthetist will leave specific instructions.
- Any further bolus doses of local anaesthetic must be administered by the anaesthetist.
- *There is no evidence to support elective instrumental delivery.*
- The patient should be informed of the puncture.
- Inform anaesthetist if the woman develops a headache.

Local anaesthetic toxicity (IV injection)

Suspect this if epidural catheter is blood-stained and epidural not effective. Features include tinnitus, tingling in the face, dizziness, confusion, slurred speech, loss of consciousness and cardiovascular collapse. If the mother has any of these during a bolus, stop the injection and call the anaesthetist. Turn mother to lateral position, give oxygen and check the vital signs.

Total spinal

Occurs when catheter is placed intrathecally.

Features: rapid onset of analgesia and dense motor block followed by nausea and vomiting, pallor and sweating, possibly leading to loss of consciousness and apnoea (cessation of breathing).

Blood pressure will be very low. Maternal heart rate may be high or low. The fetal heart will almost certainly deteriorate.

Initial treatment is as for hypotension:

- Full lateral position.
- Open drip fully.

- Oxygen by mask (may need support of breathing; check breathing and commence basic life support if needed).
- Call the anaesthetist.
- Have ephedrine and cardiac arrest trolley ready in the room.

Dense motor block

The woman should not mobilize until motor block has worn off. The block has worn off when the mother is able to straight-leg raise, bring her knees up to her chest, and push hard against resistance with both feet, without difficulty in both lower limbs.

There should be hourly position changes, to prevent pressure-related problems. These should be continued until the motor block has worn off completely.

Bladder distension

Regular voiding should be encouraged during labour, particularly before a bolus is given and until the epidural has worn off. Distension may be palpable and/or may cause breakthrough pain. In-and-out catheterization should be performed if the mother is unable to void spontaneously.

Call the anaesthetist if any of the following occurs:
    Inadequate anaesthesia
    Hypotension
    Headache following dural tap
    Symptoms of local anaesthetic toxicity – see previous page
    Dense motor block
    Any other concern

Discontinuation of epidural:

- After delivery, remove the catheter with a gentle, steady pull, ideally with the woman in the same position as during insertion. The tip of the catheter should be checked for completeness and a record made.
- Before removing catheter, always check whether LMWH (Fragmin) was given. If LMWH has been given, at least 12 hours must elapse before the cathter is removed.
- The woman should not be allowed to mobilize until she is able to flex both hips and knees against resistance. She should be accompanied when she first walks.

Repair of episiotomy and first-/ second-degree perineal tear

Indications for episiotomy include:

- preventive action when perineal tear is imminent
- to expedite delivery in cases of fetal distress or maternal exhaustion
- instrumental delivery
- shoulder dystocia.

Both the indication for episiotomy and consent must be documented in the labour records. A right mediolateral incision should be used (a midline incision increases the danger of damage to the anal sphincter).

Midwives who have been instructed in perineal repair may undertake the suturing of first- and second-degree tears and episiotomies using 2/0 Vicryl Rapide as suture material. The perineum is infiltrated with 1% lignocaine, the total amount not exceeding 20 ml.

Episiotomies should be repaired as soon as possible after completion of the third stage and preferably by the person who has delivered the baby. Subcuticular suturing is preferable to interrupted suturing of the perineal skin.

See p. 110 for guidelines on the repair of perineal tear.

The following should be documented:

☐ Type of suture.
☐ Vaginal and rectal examination at end of procedure.
☐ Swabs, sharps and instruments counted at end of procedure, and are complete.

Management of second stage of labour

Once the second stage has been diagnosed, the woman should not be left without a midwife in attendance.

The woman should be encouraged to give birth in the position she finds most comfortable.

Regardless of whether it is a normal delivery or an instrumental delivery, only the accoucheur and no more than one assistant should be at the lower end of the woman's body.

Fetal heart rate should be recorded at least after every second contraction. Blood pressure should be recorded half-hourly if normal, but every 15 minutes in hypertensive women.

 Always be certain that the cervix is fully dilated.

Duration

The median duration is 45–50 minutes in nullipara and 15–20 minutes in multipara. However, there is no evidence to suggest that the imposition of an upper time limit for duration of the second stage improves the outcome for mother or baby. More important than the time factor are evidence of progressive descent and maternal and fetal wellbeing.

- *Passive phase:* labour that is progressing normally may be in the passive stage for one hour. If the vertex is not visible within the hour, then a vaginal examination should be performed.
- *Active phase:* the registrar should be informed if the baby has not been delivered after one hour of pushing in a nullipara or after half an hour in a multipara.

Immediate versus delayed pushing

A nulliparous woman with epidural analgesia may start pushing within an hour of full cervical dilatation (immediate pushing) or after up to two hours in the passive phase (delayed pushing).

Random-allocation trials of immediate versus delayed pushing do not show a significant difference in rates of operative delivery, faecal incontinence or anal sphincter injury.

Encourage active pushing when:

- the woman has a desire to push and the vertex is visible on gently parting the labia
- one hour has elapsed since full dilatation was confirmed, and the presenting part is below the plane of the ischial spines.

Vaginal examination in second stage:

Repeat after 30 minutes of pushing, or where there is concern (eg cord prolapse)

Steady progress should be made in the active stage. Keep the team leader informed. Progress must be assessed by abdominal as well as vaginal examination (see p. 24).

Delayed second stage

Inform the registrar if:

- after one hour in the passive phase, the presenting part is not visible
- a nulliparous woman is undelivered after one hour of active pushing
- a multiparous woman is undelivered after half an hour of active pushing.

Management:

☐ Exclude disproportion. Excessive caput and moulding are indicative of obstruction.

☐ If contractions inadequate and there are no contraindications, commence Syntocinon infusion. Contraindications include disproportion, abnormal CTG, possible rupture of scar.

☐ Evaluate for instrumental delivery (see p. 177)

Situation to be avoided:

'In the second stage it is common to see assistants crowding at the lower end of the woman's body, anxiously watching her vulva as if waiting for luggage to appear in an airport carousel'

– Shelia Kitzinger, Birth and violence against women – generating hypotheses from women's accounts of unhappiness after childbirth. In: Roberts H (ed). *Women's Health Matters*. London: Routledge, 1992, Chapter 4

Management of third stage of labour

Active management of the third stage of labour reduces significantly the risk of PPH, regardless of the posture of the mother or the experience of the midwife, but there is a slight increase in the incidence of nausea and vomiting.

Active management is the recommended practice unless the mother makes an informed choice to have physiological management. The mother's choice should be documented clearly on her birth plan and labour record.

A combination of active and physiological management is unacceptable.

Physiological management is contraindicated in the following circumstances:

- operative delivery
- induced or augmented labour
- polyhydramnios
- previous postpartum haemorrhage
- epidural analgesia
- diabetes mellitus
- prolonged labour
- multiple pregnancy
- antepartum haemorrhage
- anticoagulant therapy
- anaemia
- grandmultiparity.

Active management

1. Give oxytocic drug with delivery of the anterior shoulder. IM Syntometrine 1 ml to the upper thigh muscle is the drug of choice unless contraindicated (see below), in which case give IM Syntocinon 10 IU.

Contraindications to Syntometrine:

- hypertension, pre-eclampsia
- severe cardiac disease
- pulmonary oedema
- hepatic or renal impairment.

2. Clamp the cord early (within 1–3 minutes of birth).

3. Deliver placenta and membranes by controlled cord traction with next uterine contraction.

If not delivered within 20 minutes, refer to obstetrician.

Physiological management

- Give no oxytocic drug.
- Leave cord to pulsate; do not clamp or cut.
- Careful watching and waiting. No cord traction.
- Encourage breastfeeding.
- Observe for signs of separation: lengthening of cord, gush of blood, rise of uterine fundus.
- Encourage maternal effort aided by gravity.
- *If not delivered within one hour (earlier if there is concern regarding blood loss or maternal condition), then refer to obstetrician.*

Care of the newborn

 For the majority of infants, the needs after delivery are a warm welcome, clear airways, and vigilance.

No benefits have been demonstrated for the routine suctioning of the newborn's oral and nasal passages. However, if there has been any indication of meconium-stained amniotic fluid, then the paediatrician should be called to delivery and the airways cleared under direct vision. The oropharynx should always be cleared before the nasal passages.

Vitamin K

Information regarding the use of vitamin K should be given to all mothers. Valid parental consent should be obtained and documented.

Routes of administration:

- *Intramuscular:* vitamin K 1 mg IM. Inexpensive and easy to administer. There has been some concern about possible links with childhood cancer, but further studies have found no link between vitamin K and cancer. Parenteral injection in premature babies is associated with an increased risk of kernicterus, so babies weighing less than 1500 g should receive the lower dose of 0.5 mg IM.
- *Oral:* Konakion MM Paediatric (Roche) is licensed for this indication. Dose 2 mg at birth and 2 mg within the next seven days. For breastfed babies, a further 2-mg dose is given at one month; this dose is omitted in formula-fed babies because formula feeds contain vitamin K.

Standard practice is to use the injectable vitamin K preparation. Where parents opt for the oral preparation, refer to patient group direction

If oral vitamin K has been chosen by a breastfeeding mother, then adequate arrangements should be made between the midwife, health visitor, GP and parents to ensure that the third dose is given at one month.

Vitamin K is indicated particularly in babies of women who have taken anticonvulsants (eg phenytoin) or oral anticoagulants in pregnancy.

Identification of the baby

The delivering/supervising midwife is responsible for the correct labelling of the baby before leaving the labour ward.

An identifying band should be attached securely to each ankle of the baby. This should be done in the presence of the mother if possible. The baby's name and the mother's hospital number should be written clearly on each band.

Prevention of hypothermia

Hypothermia is a core temperature of less than 35°C. Heat loss is more rapid and consequences are more severe in immature babies.

The ideal delivery-suite environment for a baby is:

- still air
- temperature 34°C
- 100% relative humidity.

Therefore:

- optimize temperature
- ensure room is not draughty.
- dry baby at birth and wrap in a dry towel
- if resuscitation is required, use resuscitaire (ie place baby under radiant heat).

Management of hypoglycaemia

Hypoglycaemia is a blood glucose level of <2.7 mmol/l.

The following are associated with increased risk of hypoglycaemia:

- preterm
- small for gestational age (below third centile)
- macrosomia
- diabetic mother
- hypothermia.

Signs include cold, sweatiness, jitteriness, behaviour changes, floppiness, apnoea, cyanosis and pallor. Babies with any of these signs should have their blood glucose measured.

Urgent action is required:

☐ Inform paediatrician.
☐ Give dextrose as prescribed by paediatrician. Baby may have to be transferred to special-care baby unit.

Preventive care

Babies small for gestational age, and other babies at increased risk, should have:

- early feeding (within two hours of delivery)
- regular feeding (three-hourly)
- blood glucose checked (dipstick) before each feed in first 48 hours.

Criteria for paediatric attendance at delivery

If any of the following are noted, a paediatrician must be called to attend the delivery:

- fetal distress
- abnormal presentation
- prolapsed cord
- antepartum haemorrhage
- meconium-stained amniotic fluid
- forceps/ventouse delivery (except lift-out procedures, where there is no fetal distress)
- caesarean section if performed under general anaesthesia or if there is a fetal indication (such as intrauterine growth restriction)
- severe pre-eclampsia
- drug abuse/addiction by mother
- diabetes mellitus
- multiple pregnancy
- breech vaginal delivery
- preterm delivery (<36 weeks)
- Rhesus isoimmunization
- fetal hydrops
- polyhydramnios
- congenital abnormalities
- anticipated shoulder dystocia
- concern of attending midwife/obstetrician

In the case of prolonged rupture of membranes (>24 hours), ear and umbilical swabs should be obtained from the baby and the paediatrician should be informed.

The midwife or obstetrician should use their clinical judgement to determine whether to call the first on-call or second on-call paediatrician, depending on the degree of risk.

Meconium-stained amniotic fluid

Risk to baby: meconium aspiration syndrome. The risk is more significant when there is thick meconium.

When there is thick meconium, amnio-infusion should be considered as it is associated with improved perinatal outcome. About 500 ml of normal saline at room temperature is infused via a transcervical tube (intrauterine catheter or nasogastric tube) at 15 ml/min.

In labour

- [ ] Inform paediatrician.
- [ ] Prepare resuscitaire and endotracheal tubes.
- [ ] CTG.

At vaginal delivery

On delivery of the head, suck mouth and nostrils to remove particulate material. Avoid deep suction.

If baby is pink, vigorous and not in respiratory distress, then no further resuscitation is necessary.

If baby is floppy at birth, then visualize the vocal cord and suck if necessary.

If no meconium is seen below cord and Apgar score at five minutes is greater than 8:

- Observe on postnatal ward – respiration, feeding, finger-prick glucose.
- Review by paediatrician at one to two hours.
- Observe for 12–24 hours.

Admit into SCBU for observation if

- meconium is seen below cord
- there is respiratory distress
- baby is still floppy at five minutes.

If the mother has had pethidine in the last four hours, give naloxone to baby and observe for 10 minutes. If the baby is still floppy, admit to SCBU.

Check cord blood gases.

At caesarean section

Transfer immediately to resuscitaire. Principles are then the same as above.

Neonatal resuscitation

All midwives, obstetricians and paediatricians have a responsibility to achieve and maintain skills needed for neonatal resuscitation.

A list of equipment and drugs is kept in the delivery rooms, obstetric theatre and on resuscitaires.

All delivery rooms, obstetric theatres and resuscitaires must be checked daily and before use.

All equipment and drugs used during resuscitation must be replaced as soon as possible.

Heaters should be turned on and warm towels should be readily available.

Principles

At the onset of acute hypoxia fetal breathing movements become more rapid. As the oxygen levels continue to fall, the regular breathing movements cease as the centres responsible for controlling them are unable to function due to lack of oxygen. The fetus enters a period known as **primary apnoea**. The heart rate falls but the blood pressure is maintained.

If the hypoxia continues and the fetus is not delivered, gasping activity begins. As the gasps fail to aerate the lungs, they fade away. This is because increasing acidosis and hypoxia interfere with the ability of the heart muscle to function effectively. The gasps eventually cease and the fetus enters **secondary** or **terminal apnoea**.

Infants in primary apnoea will quickly recover if the airway is open and oxygenated blood is transported to the heart and lungs. If the infant is in terminal apnoea, he/she will not recover without intervention and may die despite receiving help. It is not possible to distinguish if an infant who is not breathing at birth is in primary apnoea and about to gasp, or whether he/she has taken his last gasp *in utero* and is now in terminal apnoea.

 All infants born apnoeic must be presumed to be in terminal apnoea.

Avoid thermal stress

Keep the baby dry and warm: all infants must be dried thoroughly and wrapped in clean, warm towels. Cold stress increases metabolic acidosis.

Airway

Ensure clear airway: the correct position for an infant for *all* resuscitation procedures is the neutral position. Both hyperextension and hypoextension of the neck will obstruct the airways.

Deep suction of the airways should be avoided for at least five minutes after birth, except where there has been a history of meconium-stained amniotic fluid.

Evaluation

The following three criteria should be evaluated in order (see Figure 1):

- breathing
- heart rate
- colour.

Breathing

If the airway is clear and effective breathing has not been established it will be necessary to provide oxygenation by means of assisted breaths. Weak respiratory efforts should be considered the same as no respiratory effort. Provide *five* inflation breaths to clear lung fluid. These are assisted breaths of about 30 cm H_2O for about 2–3 seconds. Once inflation breaths have been given, reassess the heart rate and colour. If the heart rate is increasing and in the infant is pink, you have successfully inflated the lungs.

Reassess if effective breathing has not been established and/or the infant is not pink:

- Check the infant's airway.
- Is there chest movement when you provide ventilatory breaths?

Cardiac compression

In this event, cardiac compression will be necessary to support circulation until effective oxygenation and pulmonary blood flow are established.

Call for help (paediatric assistance bleep . . .).

- Grip the chest in both hands, placing the thumbs together at the front and the fingers over the spine.
- Position the thumb in the midline just below an imaginary line joining the nipples.
- Aim to halve the distance between the sternum and the spine.

- Pause briefly between each compression. Aim for 40–60 compressions/ minute.
- Reassess heart rate every 30 seconds. Continue compression until pulse rate is 80/minute.
- Conventional ratio is three compressions to one breath.
- If there is no response to adequate compression and lung inflation, it may be necessary to use drugs. Usually drugs are required only in the most critically distressed infant.
- Midwives may administer only vitamin K and naloxone (patient group directions).
- Check umbilical cord blood gases.

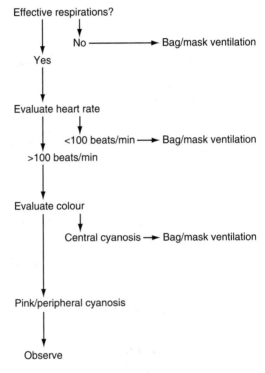

Figure 1   *Response to evaluation*

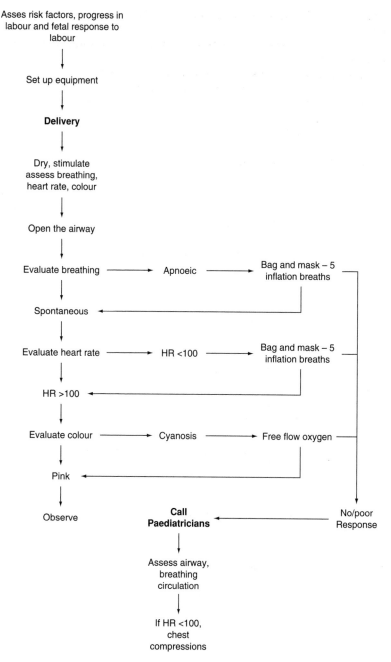

Figure 2 *Algorithm for neonatal resuscitation*

Babies born before arrival at hospital

Babies born before arrival at hospital have relatively high morbidity rates due to immaturity and low birth weight. The main risk, irrespective of birth weight, is hypothermia.

Some deliveries without medical or midwifery assistance take place at home. These should be managed according to local protocol, and transfer to hospital is not always necessary. Others will happen on the way to hospital or elsewhere outside the home.

There may be background psychosocial problems and these should be addressed where possible. In some cases, the pregnancy has been concealed or there has been no antenatal care.

Mother

☐ Placenta delivered, complete?
☐ Uterus firmly retracted?
☐ Postpartum haemorrhage?
☐ Genital tract lacerations needing repair?
☐ Blood pressure, pulse, temperature.
☐ Any obstetric, medical or social problems?

Baby

☐ Ensure baby is warm.
☐ Check colour, breathing, heart rate; call paediatrician if indicated.
☐ Birth weight.
☐ Administer vitamin K, with mother's consent.

Woman with a history of childhood sexual abuse

General measures

- Give reassurance.
- Provide the woman with a sense of control.
- Assure her that you will respect her wishes.
- The presence of a support person can be very helpful.

Communication

Choose your words carefully. Words such as 'relax' and 'luv' may bring back sad memories. Maintain confidentiality.

Physical examination

- Minimize internal examinations.
- Find out if anything could be done to make it less stressful, eg the woman may wish to take up a particular position or avoid the dorsal position.
- Let the woman know that she can stop the procedure or examination at any time if she finds it too uncomfortable.

Handle the following with extra sensitivity:

- performing episiotomy
- repairing episiotomy or tear
- lithotomy position.

Flashbacks

These may manifest as a panic attack, hyperventilation, a facial expression or a subtle change in body language. Be alert to non-verbal cues.

Use of birthing pool

Women using the birthing pool should be looked after only by midwives who have acquired the requisite skills and confidence.

Inclusion criteria

☐ 37 completed weeks.
☐ Normal pregnancy.
☐ Singleton fetus with cephalic presentation.
☐ No systemic sedation.
☐ Spontaneous rupture of membranes <24 hours.
☐ Normal observations: pulse, temperature, blood pressure.
☐ Normal CTG.

Exclusion criteria

- antepartum haemorrhage
- induction of labour
- meconium-stained amniotic fluid
- intrauterine growth restriction
- multiple pregnancy
- malpresentation
- previous caesarean section
- medical conditions such as diabetes, epilepsy
- any condition requiring continuous fetal monitoring
- mother requiring IV cannula.

Conduct of labour

The pool:

- Water depth should be such that the torso is exposed (ie not immersed), to facilitate thermoregulation through evaporation.
- Should be free of debris during delivery.
- Floor should be dry.
- Temperature not to exceed 37°C. Check temperature of pool and parturient hourly.

Analgesia: Entonox may be used. If pethidine or epidural is required, the mother will have to leave the pool.

Progress of labour:

- Vaginal examinations must be performed out of the pool.
- Progress should be recorded on the partogram.

Support in labour:

- The woman should not be left on her own at any time.
- Give liberal oral fluids and avoid dehydration.

Delivery

- Two midwives should be present at delivery.
- Do not perform episiotomy or cut cord under water.
- If the baby is delivered in water, ensure the head is the first part to emerge from water.
- Third stage, whether active or physiological, must be performed out of water.

Immediate postpartum care

It is advisable for the mother and baby to remain in the midwife's care, on the delivery suite, for one hour after delivery. If there are any deviations from normal wellbeing of the mother or the infant, then the obstetrician or paediatrician must agree transfer to the postnatal ward.

Skin-to-skin contact

Benefits:

- maintenance of baby's body temperature
- more successful breastfeeding.

The mother, regardless of whether she intends to breastfeed or formula-feed, should be encouraged to have skin-to-skin contact with the infant immediately following delivery.

Skin-to-skin contact may be delayed where there are concerns about the wellbeing of mother or baby, but it should not be delayed or interrupted by routine procedures such as weighing the baby.

For babies requiring resuscitation, skin-to-skin contact should be established once the baby has been resuscitated.

The first feed is given once the baby shows signs of readiness (sucking, rooting, hand-to-mouth movements).

Skin-to-skin contact (or refusal of) should be documented.

Care of the mother

If an epidural catheter is in place, then it should be removed before the mother leaves the delivery suite. The tip of the catheter should be checked for completeness and a record made (see p. 42).

The mother should be offered a bed bath or shower, as well as light refreshment, and made comfortable before arrangements for transfer to the postnatal ward.

Documentation

The midwife is responsible for seeing that all observations are made and recorded before transfer to the postnatal ward. Any deviations from normal should be reported to the obstetrician on duty.

- ☐ Case notes (mother and baby).
- ☐ Birth register.
- ☐ Maternity information system (computer).

Further reading

Prelabour rupture of membranes at term (37–42 weeks)

Flenady V, King J. Antibiotics for prelabour rupture of membranes at or near term. Cochrane Review. In: *The Cochrane Library*, Issue 2, 2003. Oxford: Update Software.

Shetty A, Stewart K, Stewart G, *et al*. Active management of term prelabour rupture of membranes with oral misoprostol. *Br J Obstet Gynaecol* 2002; **109**: 1354–8.

Tan BP, Hannah ME. Prostaglandins versus oxytocin for prelabour rupture of membranes at or near term. Cochrane Review. In: *The Cochrane Library*, Issue 2, 2003. Oxford: Update Software.

Management of first stage of labour

Albers LL, Anderson D, Cragin L, *et al*. The relationship of ambulation in labor to operative delivery. *J Nurse Midwifery* 1997; **42**: 4–8.

Andrews CM, Chrzanowski M. Maternal position, labour and comfort. *Appl Nurs Res* 1990; **3**: 7–13.

Caldeyro-Barcia R, Noriega-Guerra L, Cibils LA, *et al*. Effect of position changes on the intensity and frequency of uterine contractions during labor. *Am J Obstet Gynecol* 1960; **80**: 284–90.

Cassidy P. Management of the first stage of labour. In: Bennett VR, Brown L (eds). *Myles' Textbook for Midwives*. London: Churchill Livingstone, 1999, p. 414.

Hodnett ED. Caregiver support for women during childbirth. Cochrane Review. In: *The Cochrane Library*, Issue 2, 2003. Oxford: Update Software.

Newton C, Beere P. Oral intake in labour: Nottingham's policy formulated and audited. *Br J Midwifery* 1997; **5**: 418–22.

O'Sullivan G. The stomach: fact and fantasy: eating and drinking during labour. *Int Anesthesiol Clin* 1994; **32**: 31–44.

Pengelley L, Gyte G. Eating and drinking in labour (V): an update of the NCT briefing paper. *Pract Midwife* 1998; **1**: 26–8.

Fetal monitoring

Gibb D, Arulkumaran S. *Fetal Monitoring in Practice*. Oxford: Butterworth-Heinemann, 1992. (For procedure for prolonged bradycardia, see p. 110.)

K2 Medical Systems. Fetal Monitoring Training System (software). Plymouth; K2 Medical Systems. www.k2ms.com

McIntosh MCM. Continuous fetal heart rate monitoring: is there a conflict between confidential enquiry findings and results of randomised trials? *J R Soc Med* 2001; **94**:14–16.

National Institute for Clinical Excellence. *Clinical Guideline C. The Use of Electronic Fetal Monitoring*. London: National Institute for Clinical Excellence, 2001.

Royal College of Obstetricians and Gynaecologists. *The Use of Electronic Fetal Monitoring*. London: Royal College of Obstetricians and Gynaecologists, 2001.

Fetal scalp blood sampling

Gibb D. Intrapartum care. In: Clements RV (ed). *Risk Management and Litigation in Obstetrics and Gynaecology*. London: RSM Press, 2001, pp. 167–203.

Augmentation of labour

Cheek TG, Samuels P, Miller F, *et al*. Normal saline i.v. fluid decreases uterine activity in active labour. *Br J Anaesth* 1996; **77**: 632–5.

Fraser WD, Turcot L, Krauss I, Brisson-Carrol G. Amniotomy for shortening spontaneous labour. Cochrane Review. In: *The Cochrane Library*, Issue 3, 2002. Oxford: Update Software.

Kuller R, Hofmeyr GJ. Tocolytics for suspected intrapartum fetal distress. Cochrane Review. In: *The Cochrane Library*, Issue 3, 2002. Oxford: Update Software.

Epidural analgesia in labour

Association of Anaesthetists of Great Britain and Ireland and Obstetric Anaesthetists' Association. *Guidelines for Obstetric Anaesthesia Services*. London: Association of Anaesthetists of Great Britain and Ireland and Obstetric Anaesthetists' Association, 1998.

Fernando R, Price CM. Regional analgesia for labour. In: Collis R, Plaat F, Urquhart J (eds). *Textbook of Obstetric Anaesthesia*. London: Greenwich Medical Media, Chapter 6, pp. 71–97.

Gaiser RR, Venkateswaren P, Cheek TG, *et al*. Comparison of 0.25% ropivacaine and bupivacaine for epidural analgesia for labor and vaginal delivery. *J Clin Anesth* 1997; **9**: 564–8.

Hofmeyr GJ. Prophylactic intravenous preloading for regional analgesia in labour. Cochrane Review. In: *The Cochrane Library*, Issue 2, 2003. Oxford: Update Software.

Horlocker TT, Heit JA. Low molecular weight heparin: biochemistry, pharmacology, perioperative prophylaxis regimens, and guidelines for regional anaesthetic management. *Anesth Analg* 1997; **85**: 874–85.

Litwin AA. Mode of delivery following labor epidural analgesia: influence of ropivacaine and bupivacaine. *Am Assoc Nurse Anest J* 2001; **69**: 259–61.

Management of second stage of labour

Cardozo LD, Gibb DMF, Studd JWW *et al*. Predictive value of cervimetric labour patterns in primigravidae. *Br J Obstet Gynaecol* 1982; **89**: 33–8.

Fitzpatrick M, Harkin R, McQuillan K *et al*. A randomised clinical trial comparing the effects of delayed versus immediate pushing with epidural analgesia on mode of delivery and faecal continence. *Br J Obstet Gynaecol* 2002; **109**: 1359–65.

Fraser WD, Marcoux S, Krauss I *et al*. Multicenter, randomized, controlled trial of delayed pushing for nulliparous women in the second stage of labor with continuous epidural analgesia. The PEOPLE (Pushing Early or Pushing Late with Epidural) Study Group. *Am J Obstet Gynecol* 2000; **182**: 1165–72.

Gibb DMF, Cardozo LD, Studd JWW *et al*. Outcome of spontaneous labour in multigravidae. *Br J Obstet Gynaecol* 1982; **89**: 708–11.

Gupta JK, Nikodem VC. Position for women during second stage of labour. Cochrane Review. In: *The Cochrane Library*, Issue 2, 2003. Oxford: Update Software.

Maresh M, Choong KH, Beard RW. Delayed pushing with lumbar epidural analgesia in labour. *Br J Obstet Gynaecol* 1983; **90**: 623–7.

Saunders NJ, Spiby H, Gilbert L, *et al*. Oxytocin infusion during second stage of labour in primiparous women using epidural analgesia: a randomised double blind placebo controlled trial. *Br Med J* 1989; **299**: 1423–6.

Stewart KS. The second stage. In Studd J (ed), *Progress in Obstetrics and Gynaecology*, Volume 4. Edinburgh: Churchill Livingstone, 1984, pp. 197–216.

Vause S, Congdon HM, Thornton JG. Immediate and delayed pushing in the second stage of labour for nulliparous women with epidural analgesia: a randomised controlled trial. *Br J Obstet Gynaecol* 1998; **105**: 186–8.

Repair of episiotomy and first-/second-degree perineal repair

Kettle C, Johanson RB. Absorbable synthetic versus catgut suture material for perineal repair. Cochrane Review. In: *The Cochrane Library*, Issue 2, 2003. Oxford: Update Software.

Kettle C, Johanson RB. Continuous versus interrupted sutures for perineal repair. Cochrane Review. In: *The Cochrane Library*, Issue 2, 2003. Oxford: Update Software.

Management of third stage of labour

McDonald S. Physiology and management of the third stage of labour. In: Bennett VR, Brown L (eds). *Myles' Textbook for Midwives*. London: Churchill Livingstone, 1999. p. 476.

Prendiville WJ, Elbourne D, McDonald S. Active versus expectant management in the third stage of labour. Cochrane Review. In: *The Cochrane Library*, Issue 2, 2003. Oxford: Update Software.

Rogers J, Wood J, McCandish R, *et al*. Active versus expectant management of the third stage of labour: the Hinchingbrooke randomised controlled trial. *Lancet* 1998; **351**: 693–9.

Immediate postpartum care

Anderson GC, Moore E, Hepworth J, Bergman N. Early skin-to-skin contact for mothers and their healthy newborn infants. Cochrane Review. In: *The Cochrane Library*, Issue 2, 2003. Oxford: Update Software.

Christensson K, Siles C, Moreno L, *et al*. Temperature, metabolic adaptation and crying in healthy full-term newborns cared for skin-to-skin or in a cot. *Acta Paediatr* 1992; **81**: 488–93.

Care of the newborn

Dear P, Newell S. *Neonatology for the MRCOG*. London: RCOG Press, 1996.

Royal College of Midwives. Vitamin K. Position paper no. 13b. London: Royal College of Midwives, 1999.

Neonatal resuscitation

International Liaison Committee on Resuscitation. Neonatal resuscitation. *Resuscitation* 2000; **46**: 401–16.

Royal College of Paediatrics and Child Health, Royal College of Obstetricians and Gynaecologists. *Resuscitation of Babies at Birth*. London; BMJ Publishing Group, 1997.

Smith CM, Watkins RC. Resuscitation of the newborn. *Curr Obstet Gynaecol* 2003; **13**:134–41.

Meconium-stained amniotic fluid

Hofmeyr GJ. Amnioinfusion for meconium-stained liquor in labour. Cochrane Review. In: *The Cochrane Library*, Issue 2, 2003. Oxford: Update Software.

Houlihan CM, Knuppel RA. Meconium-stained amniotic fluid. Current controversies. *J Reprod Med* 1994; **39**: 888–98.

Babies born before arrival at hospital

Bhoopalam PS, Watkinson M. Babies born before arrival at hospital. *Br J Obstet Gynaecol* 1991; **98**: 57–64.

Spillane H, Khalil G, Turner M. Babies born before arrival at the Coombe Women's Hospital, Dublin. *Ir Med J* 1996; **89**: 146.

The woman with a history of childhood sexual abuse

Rhodes N, Hutchinson S. Labor experiences of childhood sexual abuse survivors. *Birth* 1994; **21**: 213–20.
Tidy H. Care for survivors of childhood sexual abuse. *Mod Midwife* 1996; **6**: 17–19.

Use of birthing pool

Royal College of Midwives. The use of water in labour and birth. Position paper no. 1a. London: Royal College of Midwives, 2000.
Steer PJ, Deans AC. Labour and birth in water: temperature of pool is important. *Br Med J* 1995; **311**: 390–91.

Section 3: Abnormal and high-risk labour

'..."high risk" obstetrics...need planning, beginning in the antenatal clinic. On admission, there is further opportunity to assess risk factors but it may be more difficult later in labour when events move fast'

– Clements RV. Risk management in obstetrics and gynaecology. In: Clements RV (ed) *Risk Management and Litigation in Obstetrics and Gynaecology*. London: RSM Press, 2001, p. 96

Part I: Powers, passenger, passage

Caesarean section

Elective caesarean section

- Book with labour ward no later than 1700 the day before surgery.
- Maximum two cases per morning session (unless there is a dedicated elective caesarean section list).
- If patient falls in to any of the following categories, book for a session covered by consultant anaesthetist:
    - previous anaesthetic complications
    - obesity (body mass index >30 at booking)
    - multiple pregnancy
    - placenta praevia
    - hypertensive disease
    - diabetes mellitus
    - Jehovah's Witness
    - significant coexisting disease (cardiac/renal/respiratory).
- Low-risk patients can be admitted on the day of operation, but bloods and consent must be obtained in clinic, ranitidine prescribed, and the patient told to starve from midnight.

It is mandatory for the woman to fast for at least six hours before an elective caesarean section.

☐ Ranitidine 150 mg orally on the night of admission and at 0730 the following day.

☐ Procedure performed with the patient in a left lateral tilt.

☐ Prophylactic antibiotics should be given after clamping the cord: IV cefuroxime 750 mg (if sensitive to this, give erythromycin 1 g).

Emergency caesarean section

☐ Contact consultant on duty/call (in their absence, contact any other consultant).

☐ Classify and document the urgency of the operation (see classification on the next page).

Notify:

☐ Operating department assistant (ODA).

☐ Anaesthetist (specify the urgency of the operation).

☐ Paediatrician.

☐ Full blood count, group-and-save or cross-match as required.

☐ Obtain consent.
☐ Discontinue Syntocinon infusion, if in progress.
☐ Ensure thromboprophylaxis is administered.
☐ Check whether ranitidine was given in labour (oral ranitidine 150 mg is effective if given at least 60 min before caesarean section). If not, give ranitidine 50 mg in 20 ml normal saline iv, over 2 minutes.
☐ Catheterize the bladder.
☐ Check fetal heart tones in theatre.
☐ Anaesthetize and deliver the patient in the left lateral tilt.
☐ Cord pH should be performed following caesarean section for fetal distress.
☐ Prophylactic antibiotics should be given after clamping the cord: IV cefuroxime 750 mg ± metronidazole 500 mg (if sensitive, give erythromycin 1 g).

Classification for urgency of caesarean section

■ *Emergency – to be performed immediately:*
  – immediate threat to life of woman or fetus
  – massive antepartum haemorrhage
  – cord prolapse
  – placental abruption
  – profound unresponsive fetal bradycardia
  – fetal distress (pH ≤7.20)
  – uterine rupture.
■ *Urgent:* maternal or fetal compromise that is not immediately life-threatening, eg failure to progress.
■ *Scheduled:* needing early delivery but no immediate maternal or fetal compromise, eg intrauterine growth restriction with abnormal Doppler.
■ *Elective:* at a time to suit the woman and the maternity team, eg previous caesarean section.

When caesarean section becomes a probability for a woman in labour, she should be informed and the anaesthetist should be alerted. This may allow discussion with the woman in less pressing circumstances.

Caesarean section for breech presentation (elective or emergency)

Always confirm in theatre that the presentation is still breech, preferably by means of an ultrasound scan.

Bleeps

Bleeps should not be brought into the theatre. If a bleep goes off in theatre during induction of general anaesthesia or while the patient is under regional analgesia, it could be alarming to the patient and/or her partner. There could also be breach of confidentiality when messages are passed to the doctor.

High-risk cases

A consultant should be present for caesarean section performed for the following indications/circumstances:

- placenta praevia
- placental abruption
- multiple previous caesarean section
- body mass index >35
- delivery <32 weeks
- any other potentially complicated caesarean section.

Delivery of the placenta at caesarean section

Spontaneous separation of the placenta followed by cord traction is preferable to manual removal of the placenta. Manual removal is associated with increased blood loss and postpartum endometritis.

Thromboembolism prophylaxis

All women undergoing caesarean section must have thromboembolism prophylaxis according to the protocol on p. 142.

Delayed elective caesarean section

- Keep the woman and her partner informed of events.
- If delayed by more than four hours, start an intravenous infusion.

Recovery of obstetric patients

All patients should be recovered in a designated fully staffed and equipped recovery area. They should be under continuous clinical observation for at least 30 minutes.

☐ Continuous ECG.
☐ Pulse oximetry.
☐ Blood pressure monitoring.

The following should be documented:

- level of consciousness
- pulse rate
- pain score
- blood pressure
- oxygen saturation
- respiratory rate
- blood loss from wound (and from drain, if present)
- intravenous infusions
- blood loss from vagina
- drugs administered.

The frequency of observations will depend on stage of recovery and clinical condition of the patient, but vital signs should be recorded at least every 15 minutes.

Discharge from the recovery area should be according to a protocol agreed by the anaesthetist.

Before transfer to the postnatal ward, all patients must:

- be easily rousable
- have full airway control
- have adequate pain relief
- have normal observations.

> **!** Midwifery staff deputed to look after postoperative patients should be specifically trained in monitoring, care of the airway and resuscitative procedures and should be supervised by a defined anaesthetist at all times.
>
> – UK Health Departments. *Report on Confidential Enquiries into Maternal Deaths in the United Kingdom 1988–1990*. London: HMSO, 1994.

High-dependency care

High-dependency care is indicated in the following circumstances:

- haemodynamic instability (due to hypovolaemia, haemorrhage, sepsis)
- continuous ECG required
- invasive pressure monitoring (central venous pressure, arterial line)
- acute impairment of respiratory, renal or metabolic function.

One or more of the above is likely to happen in cases of:

- major postpartum haemorrhage
- fulminating pre-eclampsia
- eclampsia
- disseminated intravascular coagulopathy
- pulmonary oedema
- cardiac failure
- cardiomyopathy
- sudden maternal collapse
- septicaemia.

All observations and results of investigations must be recorded in a high-dependency chart.

Some patients may need to be transferred to the general HDU or ICU of the hospital. This should be done in consultation with both the consultant anaesthetist and the consultant obstetrician (see also p. 13). Timely transfer to ICU is associated with a better outcome; conversely, delayed transfer has contributed to maternal death in some cases reviewed by the Confidential Enquiries into Maternal Deaths in the United Kingdom.

Failed intubation drill

There should be no more than two attempts at intubation. Repeated attempts increase the chances of aspiration. For the second attempt, use a bougie or smaller tracheal tubes and/or McCoy laryngoscope as appropriate. Failed intubation causes no harm to the mother as long as oxygenation is maintained.

☐ Call for help.
☐ Maintain cricoid pressure
☐ Woman in supine position with left lateral tilt
☐ Give oxygen via facemask.
☐ If successful, await return of spontaneous ventilation, turn patient and allow to waken.
☐ If mask ventilation is not possible, attempt insertion of laryngeal mask airway. (This may require partial release of cricoid pressure.) If successful, turn patient and allow to waken.
☐ If LMA insertion is unsuccessful and spontaneous breathing does not return, perform needle cricothyrotomy to maintain oxygenation.

Surgery should proceed only if the mother's life depends on it (for example, in cardiac arrest or massive haemorrhage). In this case, a spontaneous breathing technique via facemask or laryngeal mask should be used and cricoid pressure maintained. Sevoflurane is the inhalational agent of choice in this situation

After waking the patient, the options are regional anaesthesia, local infiltration and awake intubation.

Instrumental delivery

Instrumental delivery carries significant risks of acute and long-term complications for mother and baby. Care should be taken in selecting cases.

Indications for instrumental delivery

Indications include:

- fetal distress
- maternal distress or exhaustion
- delayed second stage of labour (see pp. 44–45)
- after-coming head at breech delivery
- elective procedure where maternal down-bearing effort is inadvisable
  - dural tap at epidural
  - maternal heart disease
  - severe pre-eclampsia
  - respiratory distress
  - detached retina.

Conditions to be fulfilled before instrumental delivery

☐ Full cervical dilatation.
☐ Bladder has been catheterized.
☐ Fetal head at or below the level of the ischial spines.
☐ Fetal head not palpable abdominally.
☐ Position of the presenting part defined clearly.
☐ Membranes must be ruptured.
☐ Adequate analgesia.
☐ Good uterine contractions.

All women having an instrumental delivery should have a left lateral tilt to prevent supine hypotension syndrome.

Communication

The woman (and her partner, if present) should be kept informed before and during the procedure:

☐ Warn that an episiotomy may be performed.
☐ For ventouse delivery, warn to expect a temporary swelling on baby's head where cup is applied.

Choice of instrument

The operator should use an instrument that they are comfortable with.

Forceps should be used where ventouse is contraindicated (see below). Forceps are also preferable if there is poor or no maternal effort (poor uterine action, too tired to push).

For occipitoposterior and transverse positions, a metal cup is preferable to a soft cup.

Ventouse delivery

Choose the appropriate cup (soft cup for low extraction; metal posterior cup for rotational extraction).

There should be no more than three attempts over a maximum period of 15 minutes. If duration exceeds this, do not apply forceps unless fetal head has descended to the pelvic outlet; proceed to CS.

In the following cases, ventouse delivery may be performed by an experienced obstetrician when the cervix is 9 cm dilated:

- delivery of the second twin
- cord prolapse
- fetal distress with the presenting part below the level of the ischial spines.

Contraindications to ventouse delivery

The following are contraindications for ventouse delivery:

- fetal thrombocytopenia
- maternal idiopathic thrombocytopenic purpura
- early preterm labour (<34 weeks)
- malpresentation (face or brow)
- cephalopelvic disproportion
- repeated fetal scalp blood sampling
- fetal head not engaged.

Caution
- Do not perform instrumental delivery unless absolutely certain of presentation, position of the fetal head, and cervical dilatation.
- Maternal deaths have been reported from cervical tear when a ventouse cup has been applied before full cervical dilatation.
- The operator must be willing to abandon the procedure if there is no descent of the fetal head.

Post-delivery

☐ Ensure instruments and swabs are accounted for.
☐ Cord blood analysis (pH and base excess).
☐ Recommend vitamin K.
☐ Analgesia, as appropriate.
☐ Full documentation.

Documentation

The following should be documented:

☐ indication
☐ anaesthesia
☐ instrument used
☐ findings on examination
☐ procedure
☐ time of commencement and completion
☐ any complications.

Trial of instrumental delivery

When there are features that suggest that vaginal delivery is feasible but could be difficult, a trial of instrumental delivery is acceptable practice, provided this is performed in theatre with ready recourse to CS if needed.

The features include prolonged labour, occipitoposterior position, presenting part at the level of the spines and excessive caput.

☐ Inform consultant before proceeding.
☐ Inform anaesthetist and paediatrician.
☐ Obtain consent for caesarean section to be performed if trial of instrumental delivery fails.
☐ CTG monitoring whilst setting up for anaesthesia/delivery, as well as during interval between unsuccessful trial and caesarean section.
☐ Cord blood analysis (pH and base excess).

Trial of vaginal delivery after caesarean section

All women with a uterine scar should have been assessed antenatally and a decision made as to mode of delivery (trial of vaginal delivery or elective CS). The guidance here applies only to a trial of vaginal delivery after one previous CS.

Action plan for trial of vaginal delivery

- [ ] Inform woman of the risk of scar rupture.
- [ ] IV access.
- [ ] Full blood count.
- [ ] Group-and-save.
- [ ] Monitor maternal pulse.
- [ ] Continuous electronic fetal monitoring.
- [ ] Exclude malpresentation.
- [ ] Offer epidural analgesia.

Once labour is established, assess cervix every three hours.

If the woman has not had a vaginal delivery previously, expect progress to follow the pattern of a primipara.

A repeat of CS is indicated when the alert line on the partogram has been crossed by two to three hours.

Use of Syntocinon

- Only with approval of senior obstetrician.
- The woman must be informed of the increased risk of scar rupture. This discussion should be documented.
- Scar rupture is more likely to occur if prostaglandin has been given.
- Dose increment at 30-minute intervals.
- Proceed to caesarean section if there is no change in cervical dilatation two hours after commencement of Syntocinon infusion.
- Be extra vigilant for signs of imminent or actual scar rupture: proceed to caesarean section if any sign is observed.

Signs of scar rupture or imminent rupture

Things to look out for include:

- maternal tachycardia
- poor progress in labour
- vaginal bleeding
- fetal distress
- sudden cessation of contractions
- reduction in intensity of contractions.

 Uterine rupture may occur without any warning signs.

Post-delivery

Transcervical palpation of the lower segment to exclude a scar rupture should be performed only if PPH occurs.

Induction of labour

The indication for induction and the patient's consent should be documented.

High-risk inductions should be commenced on the delivery suite.

Ideally, the woman would have been offered membrane-sweep before admission to the delivery suite. She should have been informed that membrane-sweeping is not associated with increased risk of infection but may cause discomfort and bleeding.

Methods

- *Prostaglandin (PGE$_2$):* if membranes intact and cervix unfavourable (os closed or score <7) for artificial rupture of membranes (ARM).
- *ARM:* if cervix favourable and membranes accessible.
- *Syntocinon infusion:* if membranes ruptured. If spontaneous rupture has not occurred, ARM should be performed before commencement of Syntocinon. Syntocinon infusion should not be started within six hours of the last dose of PGE$_2$.

For all methods:

☐ Confirm indication and gestational age; obtain consent.
☐ Exclude contraindications
   – major placenta praevia
   – abnormal lie.
☐ Commence CTG; if abnormal, inform registrar.
☐ Cervical assessment
   – cervical score (see below)
   – exclude cord presentation
   – proceed to ARM or prostaglandin induction.

Artificial rupture of fetal membranes

The midwife may perform ARM if the following criteria are met:

☐ Head is engaged.
☐ Vertex is presenting.
☐ Cord presentation has been excluded.

Contraindications to ARM are:

- abnormal lie
- cord presentation
- placenta praevia.

After ARM, check for cord prolapse and meconium-staining of amniotic fluid. Document the fetal heart rate.

Prostaglandin induction of labour

- *Gel:* see algorithms on pp. 85–86.
- *Tablets (intravaginal):* PGE$_2$ 3 mg every six to eight hours; maximum dose 6 mg for all women.

Use prostaglandin with caution in the following:

- previous caesarean section
- multiple pregnancy
- breech presentation
- compromised fetus (intrauterine growth restriction, oligohydramnios, abnormal CTG, Doppler or biophysical profile)
- previous difficult labour or delivery
- grandmultipara
- asthma or glaucoma.

Monitoring following insertion of prostaglandin

☐ CTG monitoring: if normal, discontinue after one hour but continue intermittent auscultation. If uterine contractions have not started within the hour, fetal heart rate should be recorded when contractions start.

☐ Maternal pulse, blood pressure and contractions monitored half-hourly.

☐ Woman to remain in bed for one hour after administration.

Do not:

- use KY Jelly or chlorhexidine cream during administration of prostaglandin as these delay absorption
- insert prostaglandin if you are unable to feel the cervix
- start Syntocinon within six hours of administering prostaglandin.

In cases of hyperstimulation, administer tocolysis (see p. 84).

Syntocinon infusion

Mix 10 units of Syntocinon in 500 ml compound sodium lactate (Hartmann's solution) or normal saline; with this dose, an infusion rate of 3 ml/hour = 1 milliunit/min.

Commence infusion at 2 milliunits/min (ie 6 ml/hour); increase every 30 minutes until strong, regular uterine contractions – three in 10 minutes – are obtained.

A syringe driver or infusion pump must be used.

Do not exceed 32 milliunits/min (ie 96 ml/hour) (see Table 2, p. 34).

Do not infuse through the same line as blood, plasma or insulin.

The syringe must be labelled, with the dose of drug and signatures of staff responsible on the label.

If labour is not established after five hours on this regime, then induction should be discontinued.

All women for whom labour is being induced with Syntocinon should have continuous electronic fetal monitoring.

The use of Syntocinon in the following circumstances requires the explicit approval of the consultant:

■ multiple pregnancy
■ malpresentation
■ previous caesarean section or other uterine scar
■ grandmultiparity.

Uterine hyperstimulation

This could occur with prostaglandin or Syntocinon.

Definition:

■ more than five contractions per 10 minutes for at least 20 minutes, or each uterine contraction lasting at least two minutes
■ suspicious or pathological CTG.

Management:

☐ Discontinue Syntocinon infusion.
☐ Lie on left side.
☐ In extreme cases, consider tocolysis with terbutaline 0.25 mg subcutaneously.
☐ It may be necessary to deliver the baby: is the CTG back to normal?

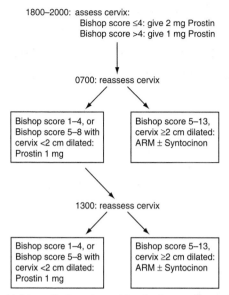

1800–2000: assess cervix:
    Bishop score ≤4: give 2 mg Prostin
    Bishop score >4: give 1 mg Prostin

0700: reassess cervix

| Bishop score 1–4, or Bishop score 5–8 with cervix <2 cm dilated: Prostin 1 mg | Bishop score 5–13, cervix ≥2 cm dilated: ARM ± Syntocinon |

1300: reassess cervix

| Bishop score 1–4, or Bishop score 5–8 with cervix <2 cm dilated: Prostin 1 mg | Bishop score 5–13, cervix ≥2 cm dilated: ARM ± Syntocinon |

If not in labour after three doses of Prostin, discuss with consultant

Figure 3   *Algorithm for cervical ripening: nullipara*

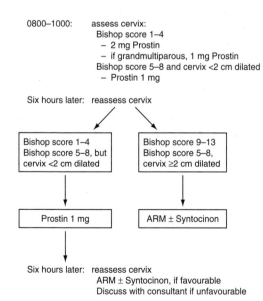

0800–1000: assess cervix:
      Bishop score 1–4
       – 2 mg Prostin
       – if grandmultiparous, 1 mg Prostin
      Bishop score 5–8 and cervix <2 cm dilated
       – Prostin 1 mg

Six hours later: reassess cervix

| Bishop score 1–4 Bishop score 5–8, but cervix <2 cm dilated | Bishop score 9–13 Bishop score 5–8, cervix ≥2 cm dilated |

| Prostin 1 mg | ARM ± Syntocinon |

Six hours later: reassess cervix
         ARM ± Syntocinon, if favourable
         Discuss with consultant if unfavourable

Figure 4   *Algorithm for cervical ripening: multipara*

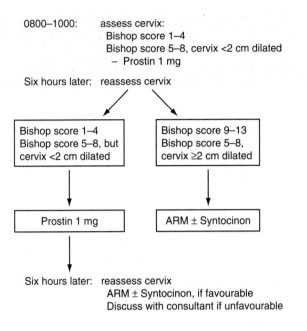

Figure 5 *Algorithm for cervical ripening: previous caesarean section*

Antenatal corticosteroid therapy

This should be given to women between 24 and 34 completed weeks' gestation presenting with any of the following:

- threatened preterm labour
- antepartum haemorrhage
- preterm prelabour rupture of membranes
- any condition requiring elective preterm delivery.

Dose: betamethasone 12 mg IM, two doses given 24 hours apart.

Note: Steroids may be given for this indication up to 36 weeks' gestation, but after 34 weeks, 94 women will need to be treated to prevent one case of respiratory distress syndrome.

Contraindications

Corticosteroid should not be given if there is any of the following:

- clinical evidence of chorioamnionitis (see p. 88)
- uncontrolled diabetes mellitus (see p. 130)
- tuberculosis
- porphyria.

Beta-sympathomimetics

The combination of steroids and a beta-sympathomimetic tocolytic poses a risk of pulmonary oedema. When this combination is used, IV fluids should be kept to a minimum and a strict fluid balance should be kept. Observe the woman for chest pain, dyspnoea and cough, and discontinue the tocolytic therapy if any of these occurs. Blood glucose and U/E should be checked every six hours.

Repeated doses

These should be given only with the approval of a consultant.

Consider the possibility of adrenal insufficiency if a woman or baby who has been exposed to repeated doses of antenatal corticosteroids has an unexplained collapse.

Preterm prelabour rupture of membranes

This is the loss of amniotic fluid per vaginum before 37 weeks in the absence of uterine contractions. (See p. 22 for management of prelabour rupture of membranes at term.)

Action plan

☐ Sterile speculum examination to confirm diagnosis and exclude prolapsed cord.
☐ Take swabs from vagina (bacteriology) and endocervix (*Chlamydia*).
☐ Full blood count, group-and-save.
☐ Midstream specimen of urine.
☐ Ultrasound scan, for presentation, fetal growth and amniotic fluid volume.
☐ Liaise with paediatrician.

Conservative management is indicated if infection is excluded and woman is not in labour.

Delivery is indicated if any of the following occurs:

- maternal pyrexia
- fetal tachycardia
- uterine tenderness
- meconium staining of amniotic fluid
- elevated C-reactive protein (CRP) and/or leucocytosis (note that steroids may elevate white cell count)
- offensive amniotic fluid
- gestation reaches 37 weeks.

Conservative management

- Alert neonatal unit.
- Four-hourly temperature and pulse rate.
- Daily fetal heart rate monitoring.
- Twice-weekly full blood count and C-reactive protein (CRP).
- Give antibiotics after initial vaginal examination:
  - erythromycin 250 mg tds for 10 days
  - *do not give co-amoxiclav as this is associated with increased risk of necrotizing enterocolitis in the newborn.*
- Betamethasone 12 mg IM, two doses 24 hours apart if <34 weeks.
- Weekly ultrasound/Doppler scan (amniotic fluid volume, fetal breathing movement).

Mode of delivery, in the absence of other complications

- *Cephalic presentation:* vaginal delivery.
- *Breech presentation:* discuss with the woman and her partner the risks and benefits of CS versus vaginal delivery.

Induction of labour

Syntocinon infusion. See p. 34 for regime. Prostaglandin may be used to ripen an unfavourable cervix (see pp. 83, 85–86) and induce labour after preterm prelabour rupture of membranes, *but*:

- insert during a sterile vaginal examination
- use only one dose.

Labour

- Continue monitoring for signs of infection (temperature, pulse).
- Inform paediatrician.
- Screen baby for sepsis.

Preterm uterine contractions

Diagnosis

- [ ] Regular contractions (at least one every 10 minutes).
- [ ] Progressive cervical effacement and/or dilatation.
- [ ] Less than 37 completed weeks of gestation.

Action plan

- [ ] Confirm gestational age.
- [ ] Assess for symptoms of urinary tract infection.
- [ ] Assess for physical or emotional trauma.
- [ ] Check temperature and pulse.
- [ ] Check for uterine tenderness.
- [ ] Assess frequency and duration of contractions.
- [ ] Assess fetal lie, presentation and station.
- [ ] Speculum examination (exclude rupture of membranes), vaginal swab and endocervical swab.
- [ ] Assess cervix.
- [ ] Midstream specimen of urine
- [ ] Full blood count.
- [ ] Urea and electrolytes.
- [ ] Kleihauer test if Rhesus-negative.
- [ ] CTG.
- [ ] If <34 completed weeks, give corticosteroid: betamethasone 12 mg IM, two doses 24 hours apart. *Note: steroids should not be used if there is clinical chorioamnionitis and should be used with caution in diabetics* (see p. 132).
- [ ] Inform consultant obstetrician.

Determine underlying cause if possible.

Consider transfer to tertiary centre (see guidelines for *in utero* transfer, p. 12).

Decide (with consultant) which of the following management options is to be followed:

- Suppress labour (but see contraindications below).
- Allow to progress to vaginal delivery (see below).
- Caesarean section, if indicated.
- Observation, if diagnosis of preterm labour is uncertain.

- [ ] Discuss with parents regarding prognosis and management.
- [ ] Inform paediatrician and neonatal unit.

Management of established preterm labour (when it is too late to suppress labour)

☐ Continuous electronic fetal monitoring.
☐ Avoid narcotic analgesia.
☐ Avoid fetal blood sampling if <34 weeks.
☐ Avoid ventouse if <34 weeks.
☐ Alert paediatrician/special-care baby unit (paediatric team to be present at delivery).
☐ Episiotomy indicated if there is delay due to head pushing against a tight perineum.
☐ Do not use 'prophylactic' forceps.

See also management of preterm breech (p. 104) and management of the pre-viable fetus (p. 94).

There is no evidence to justify routine use of prophylactic antibiotics for preterm labour with intact membranes.

Suppression of labour

Aims:

■ To enable the use of steroids for accelerating lung maturity.
■ To allow *in utero* transfer, if necessary.

Options:

■ nifedipine (unlicensed for use in preterm labour)
■ indomethacin (unlicensed)
■ ritodrine (licensed)
■ atosiban (licensed).

Ritodrine is the most widely used tocolytic, but it has many side-effects (see below).

Nifedipine is as effective as ritodrine in suppressing preterm labour and has fewer side-effects and better neonatal outcome (lower incidence of jaundice, RDS and intraventricular haemorrhage).

Indomethacin is as effective as ritodrine but is associated with premature closure of the fetal ductus arteriosus. This is more common in fetuses >32 weeks and where indomethacin has been administered for >48 hours.

Atosiban is as effective as ritodrine but has significantly fewer maternal and fetal adverse effects. However, it is substantially more expensive.

 Use nifedipine or indomethacin initially. If the response is inadequate, then a combination of both may be used. If response remains poor, or if contractions recur, then use atosiban (or ritodrine if atosiban is not available).

Contraindications to suppression of labour

Do not attempt to suppress labour if any of the following applies:

■ gestational age >35 weeks
■ cervix >4 cm dilated
■ signs/symptoms of chorioamnionitis
■ abnormal CTG
■ intrauterine growth restriction
■ placental abruption
■ bleeding (other than spotting) from placenta praevia
■ hypertension/pre-eclampsia
■ maternal thyroid or cardiac disease
■ intrauterine fetal death
■ fetal abnormality not compatible with survival.

Nifedipine

Preload with 500 ml compound sodium lactate (Hartmann's solution (because nifedipine is a calcium channel blocker and therefore lowers blood pressure).

Loading dose: 10 mg sublingually (woman bites into capsule and holds the liquid under her tongue). Repeat every 15 minutes until uterine contractions cease, up to a maximum dose of 40 mg (four capsules).

Maintenance dose: commenced six hours after loading dose. Dependent on response to initial treatment:

■ *If contractions stopped after 10 mg:* give 20 mg tds for three days.
■ *If contractions stopped after 20 mg:* give 20 mg qds for three days.
■ *If contractions stopped after 30 mg:* give 40 mg tds for three days.
■ *If contractions stopped (or still present) after 40 mg:* give 40 mg qds for three days.

After three days, reduce dose to 20 mg tds and wean off.

Indomethacin

Give as a suppository, 100 mg rectally 12-hourly for four doses.

If further doses are required after 48 hours, give 50 mg tds orally.

Do not use if there is maternal or fetal renal disease, severe oligohydramnios, or gestational age >32 weeks. If therapy continues beyond 48 hours, scan for amniotic fluid volume.

Ritodrine

Do not use if the woman:

- is diabetic
- has severe pre-eclampsia or eclampsia
- has a cardiac disease
- uses beta-agonist medication, such as salbutamol
- uses a beta-blocker
- uses a monoamine oxidase inhibitor
- is hypokalaemic.

Warn patient of the side-effects: nausea, vomiting, palpitations, sweating, hypotension and tachycardia.

Regime: add ritodrine 150 mg (ie three 5-ml ampoules) to 35 ml 5% dextrose. This gives a solution of 3 mg/ml. Administer at a rate of 1 ml/hour, using a syringe pump.

Increase by 1 ml/hour every 15 minutes until contractions are suppressed. Do not exceed the maximum infusion rate of 7 ml/hour.

Once contractions have ceased, continue infusion at the current rate for four hours, then reduce by 1 ml/hour every 30 minutes.

☐ Monitor maternal pulse, respiratory rate and blood pressure every 15 minutes. Discontinue ritodrine if maternal pulse exceeds 140 beats/min.
☐ Use pulse oximeter.
☐ Check blood glucose every four to six hours.
☐ Monitor fluid input/output strictly.
☐ Check urea and electrolytes after 24 hours.

Watch for pulmonary oedema, which may occur rapidly. Risk factors for this complication include iatrogenic fluid overload, multiple pregnancy, concomitant use of corticosteroid and infection.

Atosiban

Loading dose: 6.75 mg IV given as a bolus over one minute. (Take a vial of atosiban 7.5 mg/ml and draw 0.9 ml; this contains the required loading dose of 6.75 mg.)

Maintenance dose: 18 mg/hour IV for three hours, then 6 mg/hour IV for 3–45 hours. (Take two 5-ml vials each containing atosiban 7.5 mg/ml concentrate. Withdraw 10 ml from a 100-ml bag of normal saline, leaving 90 ml. Add the contents of the atosiban vials to the 90 ml saline. This gives a solution of atosiban 75 mg/100 ml. Infuse this at 24 ml/hour for three hours, then reduce to 8 ml/hour.)

The infusion is discontinued about six hours after contractions have ceased. The duration of treatment should not exceed 48 hours.

Side-effects include nausea, vomiting, headache and tachycardia.

Deliveries at the lower margin of viability

Pregnancy under 22 weeks

☐ The following points should be discussed and documented:
   – only one in 100 babies will survive, and of these half will have a severe disability
   – delivery may be rapid
   – the baby may be born alive, move and/or gasp.
☐ Document the agreed management plan in the case notes.

Pregnancy over 22 weeks

The following points should be discussed and documented

☐ The baby may survive short-term.
☐ Delivery may be rapid.
☐ A paediatrician and the special-care baby unit have been informed.
☐ Give the parents an information leaflet about the very premature baby.
☐ Document the agreed management plan in the case notes.

A paediatrician should attend any birth after 20 weeks' gestation, because:

■ the baby may be born alive
■ there may have been an error in assessment of gestational age
■ a decision not to resuscitate should be made by a paediatrician, not by an obstetrician or midwife.

Post-delivery care if the baby does not survive

☐ Inform consultant obstetrician of the birth.
☐ Agree postnatal care according to the wishes of the parents and inform the GP, consultant obstetrician and community midwife.
☐ Inform antenatal clinic and parent education coordinator.
☐ Offer post-delivery support, eg link with support group (see below).
☐ Inform the woman of the potential benefits of the recommended tests and investigations, and instigate as appropriate.
☐ Offer keepsakes and photographs.
☐ Discuss funeral arrangements and issue necessary documentation.
☐ Offer the opportunity to take the baby home before the funeral, and make necessary arrangements with the funeral director.

All live births must be registered, regardless of gestational age.

Support group:

Stillbirth and Neonatal Death Society (SANDS)
28 Portland Place
London
W1B 1LY

Helpline: 020 7436 5881–10:00 to 15:00 GMT, Monday to Friday
Office: 020 7436 7940–10:00 to 17:00 GMT, Monday to Friday
Fax: 020 7436 3715

www.uk-sands.org

Multiple pregnancy

Triplets and higher-order pregnancies are normally delivered by elective CS. If the woman presents with uterine contractions, then the consultant should be informed immediately and a decision will be taken regarding the timing of delivery, depending on the frequency and strength of contractions. If the woman is in established labour, then arrangements should be commenced for an urgent CS.

The following guidelines apply to the management of *twin pregnancies*.

First stage of labour

☐ Plan of management should be stated clearly antenatally; look for plan in the case notes.
☐ On admission in labour:
   – inform registrar and anaesthetist
   – secure IV access
   – full blood count, group-and-save
   – continuous electronic monitoring of both twins (dual monitor).
☐ Recommend epidural analgesia.
☐ Examine lie/presentation of both twins, with the aid of ultrasound scan:
   – *first twin cephalic, second twin cephalic:* proceed as with normal vaginal delivery
   – *first twin cephalic, second twin non-cephalic:* anticipate normal delivery of first twin with possible recourse to CS if problems with second twin
   – *first twin non-cephalic:* recommend CS.
☐ Prepare two neonatal resuscitation units.

> **!** Ensure the CTG monitor is recording heart rate of both twins, not a duplication of one twin's heart rate – be suspicious if both traces are identical (or appear to be). Where there is doubt, application of a scalp electrode to the leading twin may be helpful.

Syntocinon may be used to augment contractions, but this must be discussed first with a senior obstetrician.

Possible scenarios in the second stage should be discussed early in labour, so the mother can prepare her mind for what may happen, eg delivery in theatre and manoeuvres to deliver the second twin. This is particularly important if the presentation of the second twin is non-cephalic. If presentation of the second twin is non-cephalic, delivery should be conducted in theatre; alternatively, in an adjacent room, with regional anaesthesia.

Second stage of labour

☐ The following must be present: experienced obstetrician, paediatrician, two midwives, anaesthetist.

☐ While the leading twin is being delivered, an assistant should attempt to stabilize the lie of the second twin.

☐ Record time of delivery of first twin. *Do not give Syntometrine.*

☐ Ensure umbilical cord is clamped properly (this is important in the case of shared fetal circulation).

☐ Confirm lie and presentation of second twin by ultrasound scan.

☐ Pelvic examination to assess presentation and descent.

Delivery of second twin:

☐ Continue CTG monitoring. As long as the trace is normal, there is no reason to be worried about the clock, but CTG abnormalities are common when 30 minutes have elapsed.

☐ Use an additional clamp to mark the cord of the second twin.

Cephalic presentation:

Confirm that the presenting part is in the pelvis. It will commonly be necessary to hold the baby's head over the pelvic brim. Perform ARM with the next uterine contraction, taking care to exclude cord presentation.

If there is a delay in re-establishing uterine contractions, start Syntocinon infusion – 10 units in 500 ml normal saline (or compound sodium lactate [Hartmann's solution]); commence at 6 ml/hour and double the rate every five minutes.

If uncomplicated vertex delivery is imminent, midwife can deliver.

Breech presentation:

Offer external cephalic version (ECV). If ECV accepted and is successful, proceed as described above for cephalic presentation. If ECV declined or attempted unsuccessfully, assisted breech delivery should be conducted by the obstetrician or a midwife skilled in the conduct of breech delivery. Before rupturing the membranes, ensure the presenting part is in the pelvis – it will usually be necessary to hold the breech over the pelvic brim. Where ECV and assisted breech delivery are both declined, CS will have to be performed. In cases of footling breech, the options are breech extraction and CS.

Lie not longitudinal:

Perform external cephalic version then proceed as described above for cephalic presentation. Alternatively, convert to breech, grasp a foot vaginally through intact membranes, and then perform ARM. An assisted breech delivery is then accomplished.

Internal podalic version followed by breech extraction may be necessary in cases of fetal distress or failed external version. This should always be performed in theatre.

If the above fails, or in the absence of an obstetrician skilled in podalic version, resort to CS.

External cephalic version:

If an Syntocinon infusion is running, it should be discontinued to facilitate ECV. It may be necessary to relax the uterus with intravenous glyceryl trinitrate or subcutaneous terbutaline.

Internal podalic version and breech extraction:

Indications:

- transverse lie
- failed ECV
- fetal distress.

Do not attempt this if membranes have ruptured.

The uterus should be well-relaxed; do not perform during a contraction, and discontinue Syntocinon infusion if one has been running. If necessary, intravenous glyceryl trinitrate (100 µg repeated at two minute intervals) or subcutaneous terbutaline 0.25 mg may be given to relax the uterus.

Preferably both feet of the baby should be grasped if breech extraction rather than assisted breech delivery is intended. If only one foot can be reached, this should be the anterior foot; if the posterior foot has been grasped, it should be rotated 180° to make it anterior – this is to avoid having the anterior buttock wedged astride the symphysis pubes.

The heel distinguishes a foot from a hand. Do not bring down a foot until the heel has been identified.

'I cannot emphasise too strongly that there is a world of difference between assisted breech delivery and breech extraction. The first necessitates only a series of simple manipulations with minimal analgesic or anaesthetic requirements. The second is – or can be – a formidable operation, with considerable danger to the fetus, and one which requires the help of full anaesthesia or major nerve-blocking procedures. Many a fetus is lost because an inexperienced medical attendant plunges into the second line of treatment when the conditions and preparations are suitable only for the first.'

– Myserscough PR. *Munro Kerr's Operative Obstetrics*, 10th edn. London: Baillière Tindall, 1982, p. 76

Third stage of labour

☐ Active management of the third stage (physiological management is contraindicated).
☐ Syntocinon infusion 40 units in 500 ml for four hours.
☐ Full examination of placenta and membranes.
☐ If twins are of the same sex, send placenta for histological examination (to confirm chorionicity).

Indications for caesarean section for second twin

■ Acute fetal distress with vaginal delivery not imminent.
■ Failure of second twin to descend into the pelvis.
■ Transverse lie with failed external version.
■ Maternal haemorrhage, with vaginal delivery not imminent.
■ Obstetrician not skilled in internal podalic version or breech extraction.

Abnormal lie in labour

This could be transverse or oblique.

- ☐ Exclude placenta praevia, ovarian cyst, uterine fibroids, other possible cause.
- ☐ CTG.
- ☐ Inform the woman of the risk of cord prolapse.
- ☐ Vaginal examination
  - exclude cord presentation
  - assess cervix
  - exclude ruptured membranes.

Intact membranes

- ☐ If there are no contraindications, discuss external cephalic version (see p. 108).
- ☐ If ECV declined or unsuccessful, proceed to caesarean section.
- ☐ Following successful version, consider artificial rupture of membranes (in theatre) plus Syntocinon.

Ruptured membranes

- ■ Avoid external version.
- ■ Exclude arm prolapse.
- ■ Deliver by caesarean section.

Caesarean section:

Obtain consent for 'caesarean section', not 'Lower segment caesarean section'.

Check before the operation whether the fetal back is inferior or superior:

- ■ if the back is superior, it is easy to reach for the baby's legs and proceed with breech delivery, but beware an arm may protrude from the uterine incision (put it back) or may be mistaken for a foot (look for the heel)

- ■ if the back is inferior, internal version usually will be required, and the breech is usually easier to bring down than the head.

For a preterm baby with the back inferior, a low vertical uterine incision should be performed.

For transverse lie with arm prolapse, a classical caesarean section should be performed.

In difficult cases, it may be necessary to relax the uterus to facilitate delivery of the baby. This can be achieved with subcutaneous terbutaline 0.25 μg or intravenous glyceryl trinitrate 100 μg.

Occipitoposterior position

This should be suspected if:

- the baby's back is difficult to feel
- fetal heart tones are heard better towards the flank
- there is significant back pain.

Confirm by vaginal examination.

To ensure rotation of the head, good uterine activity is required, so consider the use of Syntocinon if the frequency and strength of contractions are suboptimal, particularly in the nulliparous woman. This also reduces the chances of a prolonged labour.

Hands-and-knees maternal posture may influence fetal position.

Persistent occipitoposterior position

The options for effecting vaginal delivery are:

- ventouse delivery, with posterior cup
- Kielland's forceps delivery
- manual rotation:
  - lithotomy position (or left lateral)
  - adequate analgesia.

Ensure the criteria for instrumental delivery are met before proceeding with forceps or ventouse.

Malpresentation

The baby's presentation reflects the degree of flexion or extension of the head:

Full flexion	–	occiput
Full extention	–	face
Deflexed but not fully extended	–	brow

☐ Inform registrar or senior obstetrician.
☐ Group-and-save.
☐ Rule out fetal abnormalities (anencephaly, goitre, hydocephalus).

Brow presentation

The forehead is the presenting part palpable on vaginal examination. Frontal sutures, anterior fontanelle, orbital ridges, eyes and root of the nose are palpable.

May change to a face or vertex presentation, so, if in early labour, await events. If there is slow progress or secondary arrest, proceed to caesarean section. If diagnosed in advanced labour, caesarean is indicated.

Face presentation

Diagnosed by palpation of chin, mouth, nose and the orbital ridges. May be mistaken for breech presentation.

If in early labour and cephalopelvic disproportion has been excluded, then allow to progress.

In advanced labour, check whether position is mento-anterior or mento-posterior:

- If mento-anterior, vaginal delivery is feasible; allow to progress, proceed to caesarean section if progress is poor. An episiotomy will usually be required.
- If mentoposterior, vaginal delivery not feasible but there is a one in four chance of rotation on reaching the pelvic floor, so may wait and see; if persistently mento-posterior, perform caesarean section.

Where vaginal delivery is anticipated, inform the mother in advance that the baby's face may be temporarily swollen (oedema) and this may cause initial difficulties with feeding.

If there are CTG abnormalities, proceed to caesarean – fetal blood sampling is contraindicated.

At caesarean delivery, flex and rotate the head to occipito-transverse before delivery.

Compound presentation

This could be cephalic presentation with a foot or hand palpable, or breech presentation with a hand palpable (take care to distinguish between hand and foot).

Manage as normal for cephalic or breech presentation, unless there is cord prolapse.

Breech presentation

Breech presentation may be diagnosed antenatally or in labour.

For cases diagnosed antenatally, mode of delivery should be stated clearly in the antenatal records.

Vaginal delivery should be performed only by a skilled attendant.

Undiagnosed breech in labour

☐ Confirm presentation by ultrasound scan.
☐ Determine wishes of the mother regarding mode of delivery.
☐ If membranes intact, assess suitability for external cephalic version (see protocol, p. 107).
☐ Recommend caesarean section if any of the following occurs:
  – pelvis clinically small or anatomically abnormal
  – big baby (consider parity and the weight of previous babies delivered vaginally)
  – hyperextended fetal head
  – footling presentation
  – intrauterine growth restriction
  – previous perinatal death
  – bad obstetric history
  – medical problems or other risk factors.
☐ Mode of delivery should always be discussed with the consultant.

Preterm breech in labour

☐ Inform consultant.
☐ Offer epidural analgesia (prevents pushing before full cervical dilatation).

There is insufficient evidence to justify routine caesarean section for preterm breech. The decision regarding mode of delivery should be made after full discussion with the woman (and her partner, if present). The discussion should be documented.

Breech vaginal delivery
First stage of labour

☐ Discuss risks of breech vaginal delivery.
☐ Discuss epidural analgesia (prevents pushing before full cervical dilatation and facilitates delivery, but may inhibit pushing in second stage).

☐ Continuous electronic fetal monitoring. A monitoring electrode may be applied to buttock if abdominal transducer not giving a good trace.

☐ IV access; full blood count, group-and-save.

☐ Anaesthetist to be available immediately.

☐ Alert paediatrician.

☐ Explain delivery to woman and partner/relative (involving the latter is important as they will observe delivery).

☐ Artificial rupture of membranes (ARM) performed only if presenting part is applied well to cervix.

☐ Perform vaginal examination immediately after spontaneous rupture of membranes (to exclude cord prolapse).

☐ Following spontaneous or artificial rupture of membranes, observe the CTG closely for the first 10 minutes (risk of occult cord prolapse).

☐ Poor progress despite good contractions suggests that the pelvis is inadequate.

☐ Augmentation is not contraindicated. However, discuss with consultant before using Syntocinon infusion. *Do not use Syntocinon if there is secondary uterine inertia.*

☐ Fetal blood sampling (buttock) may be performed if fetal distress is suspected.

☐ Proceed to caesarean section if pH <7.25.

Second stage of labour

> **!** Consider caesarean section if delay in second stage.

☐ If the woman has not had an epidural, then delivery is better conducted in theatre, with the patient prepared for an emergency general anaesthetic.

☐ Delivery should be conducted by an experienced obstetrician or appropriately trained midwife.

☐ An anaesthetist and a paediatrician should be present.

☐ The woman should be placed in the lithotomy position and catheterized.

Allow breech to descend spontaneously. Unless the perineum is relaxed, perform episiotomy when fetal anus is seen over fourchette. Use pudendal block if no epidural.

Fetal spine usually rotates uppermost. If legs are extended, deliver these by flexion at the knee joint and abduction/extension at the hips

Encourage mother to push out breech until scapulae are visible.

■ Cover baby with a towel.
■ Pull down a loop of cord only if necessary.
■ Hold femurs with thumbs on the sacrum and other fingers on the anterior superior iliac crest (pelvifemoral grip), avoiding any pressure on the fetal abdomen.

- Run a finger over the shoulder and down to the elbow to deliver the arm.
- If arms are extended, gently rotate one shoulder anteriorly and bring arm down across the chest (Lovset's manoeuvre). The nuchal line should now be visible.

Delivery of the head

You must see the nape of the neck before proceeding with delivery of the head.

- Assistant gently lifts the leg almost to the vertical, then deliver with forceps. Caution: doing this prematurely could hyperextend the neck and cause damage to the cervical spinal cord
- Use Mauriceau–Smellie–Veit manoeuvre if delivery imminent, no time to apply forceps.
- If the head fails to engage, the baby may be allowed to hang for up to one minute until the nuchal line is visible (Burns–Marshall technique). Suprapubic pressure could also be applied to guide the head into the pelvis.

Arrest of the after-coming head:

This may be due to either entrapment behind an incompletely dilated cervix or arrest at the pelvic brim. If cervix not fully dilated, incise it at 4 and/or 8 o'clock position, taking care not to cut the baby.

For arrest at the pelvic brim, apply suprapubic pressure and/or McRobert's manoeuvre (flexion and abduction of the hips).

Caesarean section for breech presentation (elective or emergency)

Confirm by ultrasound in theatre that the presentation is still breech.

Take care with opening the uterus – scalpel injuries to the baby are more likely to happen in breech than cephalic presentation. A good-size uterine incision is required, particularly in preterm deliveries, to prevent entrapment and traumatic delivery of the baby's head

External cephalic version

External cephalic version (ECV) should be offered to all women with a breech presentation, provided that the following apply:

- gestational age ≥37 weeks
- there is no contraindication to ECV
- there is no indication for caesarean section.

Risks:

- cord accidents
- feto-maternal transfusion
- placental abruption
- rupture of uterus or uterine scar.

Contraindications:

- vaginal bleeding
- abnormal CTG
- Rhesus isoimmunization
- uterine malformation
- placenta praevia.

ECV may be performed in the following circumstances, but the mother should be informed of the increased risks:

- previous caesarean section
- previous episode of bleeding
- intrauterine growth restriction
- oligohydramnios
- pre-eclampsia.

Action plan

☐ Provide information leaflet.
☐ Obtain consent.
☐ Ultrasound scan to confirm lie and presentation, assess amniotic fluid volume and exclude placenta praevia.
☐ CTG for 20 minutes before ECV.
☐ Give a tocolytic:
    – nifedipine 20 mg orally *or*
    – ritodrine 111 µg/min IV infusion over 20 minutes
☐ No more than three attempts at ECV, over five minutes.

☐ After ECV, ultrasound scan to confirm presentation.

☐ CTG for at least 20 minutes after ECV.

☐ If Rhesus-negative, send a blood sample for Kleihauer test and give anti-D immunoglobulin 500 units (unless baby's father is also Rhesus negative).

☐ Proceed to caesarean section if the CTG is abnormal or if the procedure has provoked vaginal bleeding.

☐ Document CTG observations, tocolytic given, outcome of procedure and further care.

☐ Follow-up plan agreed:
   - *ECV successful:* follow up in antenatal clinic
   - *ECV unsuccessful:* elective caesarean section or breech vaginal delivery; document mother's/couple's decision.

If a woman has had a successful ECV, she should be monitored closely in labour as there is a higher incidence of caesarean section for various reasons.

The circumcised woman

Check notes for any special instructions.

Anticipate problems and discuss these with the woman:

- difficult vaginal examination
- difficulty in catheterizing bladder
- difficulty in applying fetal scalp electrode (if required)
- genital-tract trauma during delivery
- may need anterior midline episiotomy
- psychological distress
- post-delivery urinary retention (due to pain)
- vulvovaginal haematoma.

Respect the woman's views and cultural identity, and try not to sound patronizing.

Action plan

☐ Offer epidural analgesia: this will facilitate vaginal examination and de-infibulation.

☐ If vaginal examination is difficult or impossible, the cervix may be assessed by per rectal examination, but specific consent for this must be obtained.

☐ An episiotomy will probably be necessary; this will often be a midline anterior episiotomy in cases of infibulation.

☐ Psychological support postpartum. May need referral to psychosexual services.

 Restoring infibulation (stitching together of the labia) after delivery is illegal under the Prohibition of Female Circumcision Act 1985.

If the baby is female and the family supports female circumcision, social services should be told. Explain to the woman why this is necessary. Alert the health visitor to possible child-protection issues.

Perineal tear

The perineum should be inspected after every delivery, and the presence or absence of any tear should be documented.

Classification of perineal tears

- *First degree:* laceration of vaginal epithelium or perineal skin only.
- *Second degree:* also injury to perineal muscles, but not the anal sphincter.
- *Third degree:* disruption of vaginal epithelium, perineal skin, perineal body and anal sphincter muscles:
  - *3a:* involving <50% of the thickness of the external sphincter
  - *3b:* involving >50% of the thickness of the external sphincter; complete tear of the external sphincter
  - *3c:* internal sphincter torn as well.
- *Fourth degree:* torn anal sphincter and rectal mucosa.

All tears extending to the anal margin should be regarded as third-degree tears until proven otherwise.

First- and second-degree tears: episiotomy

See also p. 43.

Vaginal tears and episiotomies should be repaired with 2/0 Vicryl Rapide.

Infiltrate with 1% lignocaine, not exceeding 20 ml.

Care should be taken to start the repair from the apex of the tear.

Skin closure: a continuous subcuticular suture is associated with less short-term pain than interrupted sutures. Apposing but not suturing the skin is associated with less dyspareunia.

A paravaginal haematoma should be suspected if there are signs of shock after the third stage of labour in the absence of significant bleeding externally. See also p. 189.

☐ Rectal examination should be performed after repair.
☐ Swab and needle count should be performed after repair.
☐ If there is a substantial periurethral tear, insert a catheter.

Third- and fourth-degree tears

 A general anaesthetic or epidural/spinal is mandatory when there is a third- or fourth-degree tear.

Repair must be performed by an obstetrician trained to do so and must be performed in the operating theatre.

- ☐ Anal epithelium repaired with Vicryl 3/0 (Ethicon) sutures, either interrupted with the knots tied in the anal lumen or continuous submucosal.
- ☐ Internal anal sphincter repaired with 3/0 PDS (Ethicon) interrupted sutures.
- ☐ External anal sphincter repaired with 3/0 PDS sutures, using either overlapping or end-to-end technique (the only published random-allocation study showed no significant difference between the two methods; results of at least four ongoing trials are awaited).
- ☐ Reconstruct the perineal muscles (failure to do so leaves a short, deficient perineum).
- ☐ Swab and needle count.
- ☐ Give cefuroxime 1.5 g and metronidazole 500 mg IV, followed by five-day course of oral cefalexin and metronidazole.
- ☐ Prescribe
  - lactulose 10 ml tds for two weeks
  - Fybogel, one sachet bd for two weeks.
- ☐ Document extent of injury and how it was managed.
- ☐ Arrange follow-up appointment with consultant obstetrician and/or perineum clinic, according to local protocol.

Part II: Medical conditions

Heart disease in labour

Principles of management

Delivery must be planned, particularly for women with severe disease. Liaise with consultant anaesthetist and cardiologist.

Prevent heart failure – avoid factors that may increase cardiac workload, including:

- excessive physical effort
- anaemia
- infection
- hypertension.

In women with obscure febrile illness, consider the possibility of endocarditis.

Action plan

☐ Antibiotic cover: all women in labour and with a structural heart defect, prosthetic valve or a history of endocarditis must have prophylactic antibiotics
  - *undergoing caesarean section:* amoxicillin 1 g IV and gentamicin 120 mg IV (over three minutes) at induction of anaesthesia, then amoxicillin 500 mg six hours later
  - *vaginal delivery:* amoxicillin 1 g IV and gentamicin 120 mg IV (over three minutes) at the onset of labour or ruptured membranes, then amoxicillin 500 mg six hours later
  - *woman allergic to penicillin or has had more than a single dose of penicillin in previous month:* vancomycin 1 g by slow IV infusion (over at least 60 minutes) before delivery, then gentamicin 120 mg IV at induction of anaesthesia or at 8 cm dilatation.

☐ Labour in left lateral or upright position.
☐ ECG.
☐ Oxygen by mask, as required.
☐ Continuous CTG.
☐ Expedite second stage (elective forceps or ventouse).
☐ Syntocinon by slow infusion for third stage (five units in 500 ml at 125 ml/hour). *Do not give ergometrine or Syntometrine.*
☐ Offer epidural analgesia (care with fluid preloading; avoid if cardiac output is restricted).
☐ Continue high-dependency care for 24–48 hours following delivery: the most dangerous time for the cardiac patient is the first 24 hours after delivery. Women with Eisenmenger syndrome need to be in the ITU for at least seven days after delivery.

If the woman is on anticoagulants:

- avoid intramuscular injections
- involve the haematologist on call
- stop heparin at commencement of labour
- resume anticoagulants post-delivery if there is no postpartum haemorrhage.

If labour starts while the patient is on warfarin, then vitamin K should be given to the mother and to the baby at delivery.

 In patients with heart disease, avoid fluid overload, tocolytics, and local anaesthetics containing adrenaline.

Peripartum cardiomyopathy

This is a disease of unknown cause in which left ventricular dysfunction occurs in late pregnancy or puerperium. The condition is rare before 36 weeks. It is characterized by the absence of recognizable heart disease before the last month of pregnancy and the absence of a known cause of heart failure.

Diagnosis: the above, plus left ventricular systolic dysfunction on echocardiography.

 Any woman without a relevant prior history and who presents with heart failure in late pregnancy should be regarded as having a cardiomyopathy until it is proven otherwise.

Risk factors:

- advanced age
- multiparity
- African descent
- hypertension
- multiple pregnancy.

Symptoms and signs:

- breathlessness
- palpitations
- swollen legs
- tachycardia
- dyspnoea
- dysrhythmia
- signs of embolism.

☐ Call for help!
☐ Manage shock: airways, breathing, circulation.
☐ Establish iv access.
☐ Full blood count, urea and electrolytes, group-and-save.
☐ Chest X-ray.
☐ ECG.
☐ Echocardiography
☐ Salt and water restriction.

☐ Continuous electronic fetal monitoring.
☐ Involve cardiologist immediately.
☐ Inform neonatologist.
☐ Inform anaesthetist.
☐ Anticoagulant therapy and treatment of heart failure as agreed with cardiologist.

A senior clinician must decide the place, time and mode of delivery. Transfer to a high-risk centre, if feasible.

Pre-eclampsia

Pre-eclampsia remains one of the main causes of maternal mortality in the UK. Complications of pre-eclampsia include:

- cerebrovascular accident
- placental abruption
- HELLP (haemolysis, elevated liver enzymes, low platelets) syndrome
- disseminated intravascular coagulopathy (DIC)
- eclampsia
- hepatic failure
- renal failure
- pulmonary oedema
- intrauterine growth restriction.

Diagnosis

Hypertension and proteinuria, with or without oedema. However, please note that not all cases present with the classic features.

There is lack of consistency in the literature over the definition of pregnancy-induced hypertension. For practical purposes, any of the following should be regarded as hypertension:

- increase in systolic blood pressure of ≥30 mmHg and/or increase in diastolic blood pressure of ≥15 mmHg, over blood pressure taken before 20 weeks of gestation
- diastolic blood pressure ≥90 mmHg (two readings taken at least four hours apart) if measurement before 20 weeks not known
- increase in mean arterial pressure (MAP) of 20 mmHg over reading before 20 weeks
- MAP ≥105 mmHg if reading before 20 weeks not known.

Pre-eclampsia is classified as severe if any of the following are seen:

- dizziness, drowsiness, visual symptoms or epigastric pain/tenderness
- hyperreflexia
- papilloedema
- systolic blood pressure >160 mmHg or diastolic blood pressure >110 mmHg
- MAP >125 mmHg
- proteinuria: 3+ on dipstick or >3 g in 24-hour urine collection
- oliguria: <500 ml in 24 hours

- thrombocytopenia: <100×10^9/l
- creatinine >100 mmol/l
- alanine aminotransferase (ALT) >50 IU/l
- pulmonary oedema.

'Pre-eclampsia is a disease of signs....symptoms are the hallmark of imminent eclampsia' – Baskett TF. *Essential Management of Obstetric Emergencies*. 3rd edn. Bristol: Clinical Press, 1999, p. 79

- Mild pre-eclampsia may progress rapidly to severe disease.
- Fits may occur without any warning signs or symptoms.
- Fits occur more frequently postpartum than intrapartum.

Action plan

☐ Check symptoms.
☐ Check reflexes and fundoscopy.
☐ Serial blood pressure recording (see below).
☐ Urinalysis.
☐ Full blood count.
☐ Group-and-save.
☐ Urea and electrolytes and creatinine.
☐ Urate.
☐ Liver function tests.
☐ Clotting screen.
☐ 16G Venflon: Hartmann's solution 85 ml/hour.
☐ Monitor urine output.
☐ Offer epidural analgesia if platelet count >100×10^9/l.
☐ Continuous electronic fetal monitoring.
☐ Inform consultant obstetrician.
☐ Inform consultant anaesthetist.
☐ Assess fetal wellbeing: growth, amniotic fluid volume, umbilical artery Doppler.
☐ Decision whether to deliver or manage conservatively:
  – *severe pre-eclampsia:* deliver, regardless of gestational age
  – *mild/moderate pre-eclampsia at term:* deliver
  – *mild/moderate pre-eclampsia preterm:* may be managed conservatively.
☐ If delivery imminent, give ranitidine 150 mg orally immediately, then 150 mg every six hours.
☐ If <34 weeks gestation, give prophylactic betamethasone for lung maturity.
☐ Commence antihypertensive treatment (see below).

Measurement of blood pressure

Automated blood-pressure-monitoring devices are convenient for monitoring trends, but they may underestimate blood pressure. If a device is used, the readings must be checked hourly against sphygmomanometer measurements.

The sphygmomanometer cuff should be at the level of the heart, and should be of appropriate size for the woman. In women whose arm circumference exceeds 35 cm, a large cuff should be used.

Korotkoff sound V is preferable to Korotkov IV for determining diastolic pressure

Severe pre-eclampsia

- ☐ Connect ECG monitor.
- ☐ Connect O_2 saturation monitor. If O_2 saturation drops below 95%, inform registrar.
- ☐ Open a high-dependency care chart.
- ☐ Check respiratory rate hourly.
- ☐ Insert a Foley catheter, and monitor fluid balance (see p. 124).
- ☐ Commence anticonvulsant prophylaxis (see below).
- ☐ Consider insertion of central venous pressure or arterial line. If central venous pressure <5 cmH$_2$O or >12 cmH$_2$O, inform anaesthetist.

 Do not transfer to another hospital unless clinical condition has been stabilized. The blood pressure should be below 160/105 mmHg and oxygen saturation should be normal. (See also *in utero* transfer, p. 12.)

Timing of delivery should be judicious. Stabilizing the patient before CS will reduce risks, but delaying delivery could increase risks; each case should be assessed on its merits.

Second stage of labour: if the active phase lasts beyond 30 minutes, advise instrumental delivery.

Third stage of labour: give Syntocinon five units IV or IM. *Do not use Syntometrine or ergometrine.*

Watch for PPH. Note that with haemoconcentration, pre-eclamptic patients are less tolerant of haemorrhage than normotensive women: observe BP and urine output

Post-delivery

- ■ Avoid nonsteroidal anti-inflammatory drugs (NSAIDs) (eg diclofenac).
- ■ Manage on delivery suite until stable.
- ■ Maintain vigilance.
- ■ Check blood pressure hourly for the first four hours, then every four hours for 12 hours, and then every eight hours for 48 hours.
- ■ Continue antihypertensive and anticonvulsant treatment as required (see below).

Antihypertensive therapy

The aim of treatment is not to normalize blood pressure but to maintain it at a relatively safe level. If blood pressure drops too low, placental perfusion will be reduced. This is particularly stressful to the growth-restricted fetus. Aim for a MAP of <125 mmHg.

If systolic blood pressure <160 mmHg, or diastolic blood pressure <105 mmHg, or MAP 125–140 mmHg, give oral Labetalol 200 mg. Expect blood pressure to drop within 30 minutes.

If systolic blood pressure >160 mmHg systolic, or diastolic blood pressure >105 mmHg, or MAP >140 mmHg, the options are hydralazine or labetalol. Hydralazine is more widely used and has been described as 'the first-line drug of choice for management of severe hypertension' (*Why Mothers Die. Report on Confidential Enquiries into Materal Deaths in the UK, 1994–96*. London: The Stationery Office, 1998, p. 92). A recent meta-analysis generated uncertainty about the agent of first choice (Magee *et al*, 2003).

Hydralazine

- ☐ Give hydralazine 5 mg bolus IV over 10 minutes.
- ☐ Simultaneously give 500 ml Gelofusine (or other colloid) over 30 minutes (see p. 125).
- ☐ Follow with hydralazine infusion 40 mg in 40 ml normal saline, via syringe pump, starting at 5 ml/hour.
- ☐ Titrate against blood pressure as follows: double every 30 minutes until stable at diastolic of 90 mmHg or pulse rate exceeds 130; do not exceed 40 ml/hour.

Side-effects of hydralazine include tachycardia, headache, dizziness, dyspnoea and flushing. These mimic deteriorating pre-eclampsia.

 Do not use hydralazine in women with cardiovascular disease.

When tailing off hydralazine (this is usually post-delivery), halve the infusion rate every 30 minutes.

Labetalol

- ☐ Give 200 mg orally, if able to tolerate oral therapy, or a bolus of 50 mg (10 ml labetalol 5 mg/ml) IV over 10 minutes. This may be repeated at 15-minute intervals up to a maximum of four doses (ie 200 mg).
- ☐ Follow with labetalol infusion 5 mg/ml delivered via syringe pump at a rate of 4 ml/hour (20 g/hour). Double the rate every 30 minutes until blood pressure is stable and within the target range. Maximum dose 32 ml/hour (160 mg/hour).

Side-effects include headache, postural hypotension (avoid upright position for three hours after IV labetalol) and nausea.

Contraindications:

- severe asthma or obstructive airways disease
- heart block
- severe peripheral arterial disease.

Anticonvulsant treatment

All women with severe pre-eclampsia should receive anticonvulsant prophylaxis.

☐ Take two ampoules of 5 g magnesium sulphate and dilute in 30 ml normal saline. This gives 50 ml of 20% $MgSO_4$ solution or 1 g/5 ml.
☐ Give loading dose of 4 g (**20 ml**) of **20**% solution IV over **20 minutes** (a rapidly given bolus may cause cardiac arrest).
☐ Give maintenance dose by infusion pump of 1 g (5 ml) per hour.

Review hourly to ensure that:

- respiratory rate is >12/min
- urine output is >20 ml/hour
- knee or forearm jerk is present
- O_2 saturation is ≥95% on air or oxygen.

Check serum magnesium level four hours after commencing infusion.

If reflexes or respiration are depressed, stop magnesium sulphate infusion and check serum magnesium level. See below for management of magnesium toxicity.

If urine output is <20 but >10 ml/hour, then adjust treatment according to plasma creatinine level:

- *Normal creatinine (100 mmol/l):* continue infusion but check magnesium level every two hours.
- *High creatinine (100–150 mmol/l):* reduce infusion to 0.5 g/hour and check magnesium level every two hours.
- *Very high plasma creatinine (>150 mmol/l):* stop magnesium sulphate infusion. Check magnesium level at once and every two hours thereafter.

If urine output is <10 ml/hour, stop magnesium sulphate infusion.

Magnesium sulphate blood levels

- *Therapeutic:* 2–3.5 mmol/l.
- *Low:* <2 mmol/l. Increase infusion rate to 2 g/hour for 2 hours, then recheck level.
- *High:* 3.5–5.0 mmol/l. Stop infusion. Restart at half the previous rate if urine output >20 ml/hour.
- *Very high:* >5.0 mmol/l. Stop infusion. Commence ECG.

Management of magnesium toxicity

Features: Loss of deep tendon reflexes, nausea, double vision, slurred speech, respiratory arrest. In severe cases there is cardiac arrest.

If magnesium toxicity is suspected:

☐ Discontinue magnesium sulphate infusion.
☐ Check [Mg] urgently.
☐ ECG.
☐ If cardiorespiratory arrest is imminent, give 10% calcium gluconate 10 ml IV over 2–5 minutes
☐ If cardiac arrest occurs – Crash call and cardiopulmonary resuscitation.

Postpartum

Continue magnesium sulphate for 24 hours postpartum or longer if the woman is still hyperreflexic.

Continue antihypertensives until diastolic blood pressure is <100 mmHg or MAP is <140 mmHg.

Post-delivery ward round (days 0–3)

☐ Check temperature, pulse, blood pressure and respiratory rate.
☐ Check O_2 saturation. If O_2 saturation <95% or respiratory rate >25/min, request chest X-ray.
☐ Assess sensorium. Abnormal sensorium with hyperreflexia is indicative of cerebral oedema.
☐ Check fluid balance.
☐ Exclude abnormal bleeding.
☐ Full blood count and coagulation screen every eight hours for the first 24 hours.
☐ Liver function tests daily.
☐ Suspect hepatic rupture if right upper quadrant pain is persistent: arrange computerized tomography (CT) scan.
☐ Medication: do current doses of anticonvulsant and antihypertensive need to be adjusted?

Fluid management in pre-eclampsia
Principles

Problems related to excessive fluids (pulmonary oedema and adult respiratory distress syndrome [ARDS]) are much more common than those related to inadequate fluids. ARDS is the most frequent mode of death from hypertensive disorders of pregnancy.

In severe pre-eclampsia, there is an increase in systemic vascular resistance. Vasodilator therapy could reduce this, resulting in precipitate hypotension and poor end-organ perfusion. Vasodilator therapy should therefore be accompanied by a fluid load to maintain or improve organ (placenta and kidneys) perfusion.

In severe pre-eclampsia, blood pressure may be maintained despite regional blockade. Preloading with fluids (before epidural) in anticipation of hypotension may be an unnecessary risk in this situation.

Oedema mobilizes back into the circulation within 24–36 hours after delivery.

Patients with excessive haemorrhage require totally different management, including invasive monitoring in many cases.

Predelivery

- Background fluids: Hartmann's solution 85 ml/hour.
- If Syntocinon infusion has been given, the volume should be included in the calculation of fluid input.
- Correct any pre-existing fluid deficits (eg long period nil by mouth, vomiting, blood loss).
- Strict fluid input/urine output chart.
- Fluid bolus 500 ml Gelofusine or Haemaccel over 30 minutes before or at the same time as
  - loading with magnesium sulphate
  - loading with antihypertensive drug
  or if urine output <100 ml in four hours.

 Do not give any woman more than two fluid boluses, unless she is bleeding.

 Diuretics (eg frusemide 10–20 mg) are not appropriate except in pulmonary oedema.

Delivery is indicated if there is:

- pulmonary oedema
- renal failure (rising urea/creatinine)
- irreversible oliguria despite the above measures.

Post-delivery

Ensure peripartum losses have been replaced. Note that a natural diuresis occurs postpartum.

Background fluids: Hartmann's 50 ml/hour for 24 hours, then 85 ml/hour. Total fluid input in the first 24 hours should not exceed 2 l.

Replace any continuing loss. Check U/E (watch for hyponatraemia).

Look for signs of pulmonary oedema: rising respiratory rate and heart rate, O_2 saturation <95% on air, chest signs, abnormal chest X-ray. If present, give frusemide as above, whatever the urine output.

CVP monitoring will usually be required in patients with significant haemorrhage, renal failure or pulmonary oedema that does not respond rapidly to normal therapeutic measures.

Management of oliguria (<100 ml in four hours)

If the woman is hypovolaemic (see below) or bleeding, replace loss.

If the woman is not hypovolaemic (see below) and not bleeding:

- Providing there are no signs of fluid overload, give 200 ml IV fluid over 30 minutes.
- If urine output does not improve, give frusemide 10 mg IV.
- If oliguria persists, consult renal physician.

Features of hypovolaemia include dry mouth, loss of skin turgor, cold extremities, raised pulse rate, hypotension, reduced pulse pressure and raised respiratory rate.

 Tachypnoea could also be a sign of fluid overload (pulmonary oedema).

Blood transfusion

Blood transfusion may increase the intravascular oncotic pressure and cause pulmonary oedema in a woman with severe pre-eclampsia. Unless it is absolutely necessary (eg acute blood loss), transfusion should be withheld until after diuresis has occurred.

Eclampsia

Management aims to:

- control convulsions
- control blood pressure
- deliver the baby.

Beware of postpartum eclampsia (see below).

Action plan

☐ Maintain airway.
☐ Turn patient to left lateral position.
☐ Oxygen by mask (at least 10 l/min).
☐ IV line.
☐ Arrest convulsion with MgSO$_4$ or with diazepam 10 mg IV.
☐ Prevent further fits with MgSO$_4$ infusion.
☐ Treat hypertension.

MgSO$_4$ is more effective than diazepam, but for most cases fits would have been aborted by diazepam in the time it takes to prepare a syringe of MgSO$_4$. Also, MgSO$_4$ must be injected slowly – whereas in the face of fits the tendency is to do things quickly.

Anticonvulsant treatment (magnesium sulphate)

☐ Take two ampoules of 5 g magnesium sulphate and dilute in 30 ml of normal saline. This gives 50 ml of 20% MgSO$_4$ solution or 1 g/5 ml.
☐ Give a loading dose of 4 g (**20 ml** of **20%** solution) IV over **20 minutes** (a fast bolus may cause cardiac arrest).
☐ Give a maintenance dose by infusion pump of 1 g (5 ml) per hour.

Review hourly to ensure that:

- respiratory rate is >12/min
- urine output is >20 ml/hour
- knee or forearm jerk is present
- oxygen saturation is satisfactory.

If convulsions recur, give 2 g (10 ml) magnesium sulphate 20% solution over five minutes.

The maintenance dose should be continued for 24 hours after the last seizure.

Side-effects of $MgSO_4$ infusion include double vision, slurred speech, respiratory depression, loss of tendon reflexes and cardiac arrest.

If reflexes or respiration are depressed, stop magnesium sulphate infusion and check serum magnesium level. Respiratory depression should be treated with calcium gluconate 1 g IV given over 10 minutes.

If urine output is <20 but >10 ml/hour, adjust treatment according to plasma creatinine level:

- *Normal creatinine (100 mmol/l):* continue infusion but check magnesium level every two hours.
- *High creatinine (100–150 mmol/l):* reduce infusion to 0.5 g/hour and check magnesium level every two hours.
- *Very high plasma creatinine (>150 mmol/l):* stop magnesium sulphate infusion. Check magnesium level at once and every two hours thereafter.

If urine output is <10 ml/hour, stop magnesium sulphate infusion.

Magnesium sulphate blood levels

- *Therapeutic:* 2–4 mmol/l.
- *Low:* <2 mmol/l. Increase infusion rate to 2 g/hour for two hours then recheck level.
- *High:* 4–5 mmol/l. Stop infusion. Restart at half the previous rate if urine output >20 ml/hour.
- *Very high:* >5 mmol/l. Stop infusion and commence ECG.

Persistent seizures

If seizures persist despite magnesium:

- Try diazepam 10 mg IV.
- Anaesthetist may give thiopentone 50 mg IV.
- Consider intubating the patient.
- Further seizures should be managed by intermittent positive-pressure ventilation and muscle relaxation.
- If the fits are refractory a computerized tomography (CT) or magnetic resonance (MR) scan should be performed.

Controlling blood pressure

See p. 122.

Avoid precipitous drop in blood pressure.

General management

(same as for pre-eclampsia, p. 120)

- Decision must be made immediately regarding mode of delivery.
- After delivery, the woman should remain in HDU until at least 24 hours have elapsed without a fit.
- Anticonvulsant therapy should be continued until 24 hours have elapsed since last fit and she is no longer hyperreflexic.
- For fluid management, see p. 124.

! If there are focal neurological signs, CT or MRI scan of the brain should be performed.

! Alert! One woman had a seizure in hospital after a CS for pre-eclampsia at term and appeared to be making a good recovery. but was found collapsed and pulseless after being left unattended in a bath on the fourth day after delivery. *Why Mothers Die. Report on Confidential Enquiries into Maternal Deaths in the UK, 1994–96*. London: The Stationery Office, 1998, p. 39.

Diabetes mellitus

Management will depend on whether the woman is on insulin.

Details of intrapartum management will usually have been decided in the joint diabetic clinic and written in the case notes.

Induction of labour or caesarean section in a diabetic woman should be performed first thing in the morning.

Induction of labour by artificial rupture of fetal membranes

- Usual dose of insulin the evening before.
- Nil by mouth from midnight.
- 0800: perform ARM and commence insulin/glucose protocol (see below).

Induction of labour with Prostin

- Allow the patient to eat and drink.
- Usual dose of insulin until she is in established labour.
- Commence insulin/glucose protocol when in established labour.

Elective caesarean section

- Bedtime snack the night before, then nil by mouth.
- Usual evening dose of insulin, or as prescribed by diabetologist.
- Skip morning dose of insulin.
- Caesarean section in the morning (first on the list).

First stage of labour

☐ Continuous fetal monitoring.
☐ Recommend epidural analgesia.
☐ Full blood count, urea and electrolytes, group-and-save.
☐ Check urine for ketones.
☐ Two IV lines
  – *line 1:* 5% glucose + 10 mmol KCl 500 ml at 100 ml/hour through infusion pump
  – *line 2:* 0.9% saline 50 ml + short-acting insulin 50 units (ie a concentration of 1 unit/ml), via pump according to sliding scale (see Table 4).
☐ Check capillary blood glucose hourly.

Table 4 *Sliding scale insulin infusion*

Blood glucose concentration (mmol/l)	Insulin infusion rate (units/h)
≤2	0
2.1–3.9	0.5
4.0–6.9	1
7.0–8.9	2
9.0–10.9	4
11.0–16	6
>16	8

Aim to keep blood glucose concentration in the range 4–7 mmol/l.

Use separate IV access for IV Syntocinon or preloading for epidural.

Be cautious with the use of a three-way tap for glucose/insulin infusions, as inadvertent disconnection of one line could be disastrous.

 Always check that the glucose drip is working.

If there are difficulties with blood glucose control, check the following:

- Pump may not be working.
- Syntocinon may have been added to dextrose instead of saline.
- Glucose drip may not be working or may be running into tissue.

 If Syntocinon is required, it should be via saline infusion, not dextrose.

Beware of secondary arrest, in view of possible macrosomia.

If shoulder dystocia is anticipated:

- discuss this with the woman
- revise shoulder dystocia drill now.

Gestational diabetic, diet-controlled

☐ Check blood glucose on admission and then hourly
  - if blood glucose <3.9 mmol/l or labour lasts >8 hours, commence dextrose 5% infusion

     – if blood glucose >7 mmol/l, commence insulin/glucose protocol (see above). Insulin may be needed in the second stage of labour due to catecholamine surge.

☐ On the day after delivery, check blood glucose levels – preprandial, two hours after lunch, and at bedtime.

☐ Arrange glucose tolerance test at six to eight weeks post-delivery.

Preterm labour

See also pp. 88–93.

Manage according to diabetic protocol.

Ritodrine should not be used.

Dexamethasone may affect blood glucose control, so avoid if glucose control on admission is poor. If glucose control on admission is satisfactory, the effect of dexamethasone can be controlled by increasing the dose of subcutaneous insulin in consultation with diabetologist.

After delivery

Capillary blood glucose monitoring every two hours.

Gestational diabetics:

■ Discontinue insulin/glucose infusion once able to eat light diet.
■ May eat and drink normal diet without subcutaneous insulin.

Insulin-dependent diabetics:

■ Once placenta is delivered, reduce insulin dose by 50%.
■ Continue infusion until woman is able to eat and drink.
■ First subcutaneous dose of insulin should overlap IV infusion by 30 minutes.
■ Restart subcutaneous insulin on pre-pregnancy dose. If this is not known, use 30/70 soluble/isophane insulin mix twice a day with meals.

Do not transfer to postnatal ward until blood glucose levels are normal and there is no ketonuria.

Hypoglycaemic shock

 Call for help: anaesthetist, registrar in medicine.

Quick dipstick test to determine whether this is hypoglycaemia (<2.5 mmol/l) or ketoacidosis (usually, but not always, >9 mmol/l).

Manage shock: airways, breathing, circulation.

☐ Continuous electronic fetal monitoring.
☐ Give 50 ml of 50% glucose IV.
☐ Chart vital signs and O_2 saturation.
☐ Repeat finger-prick glucose every 30 minutes.

Diabetic ketoacidosis

Risk factors include infection and the use of steroids to accelerate fetal lung maturity.

Presentation: nausea, vomiting, polydipsia, dizziness, tachycardia, tachypnoea, hypotension, smell of ketones.

> **!** Call for help: anaesthetist, registrar in medicine.

Woman needs high-dependency or intensive care.

Quick dipstick test to confirm this is ketoacidosis (usually, but not always, >9 mmol/l), rather than hypoglycaemia (<2.5 mmol/l).

Manage shock: airways, breathing, circulation.

☐ Continuous electronic fetal monitoring.
☐ Chart vital signs and O_2 saturation.
☐ Blood tests: full blood count, glucose, urea and electrolytes, group-and-save, blood culture, arterial blood gases.
☐ Midstream specimen of urine for bacteriology.
☐ Urinalysis.
☐ Insert Foley catheter: monitor fluid input and urine output
☐ Insert nasogastric tube (to reduce risk of aspiration).
☐ Treat dehydration: IV infusion of normal saline.
☐ Administer insulin as advised by physician (usually a loading dose of 10 units insulin, followed by an infusion of 5–10 units/hour).
☐ Give 20–40 mmol of potassium in each litre of normal saline, over three hours.
☐ Treat infection, if present.
☐ If undelivered, determine time and mode of delivery.
☐ Alert paediatricians.

Epilepsy

Management in labour

- Reassure that most will have a normal, vaginal delivery.
- Continue usual anticonvulsant regimen during labour and postpartum.
- Pain relief as for other women in labour. Inadequate analgesia induces hyperventilation (which could trigger a fit).
- Avoid exhaustion and dehydration – these may trigger fits. Fits may also be triggered by bright flickering lights, noise, lack of sleep and emotional stress.
- Patient is not to be left on her own.
- Appropriate support in cases of congenital malformation or dysmorphic features.
- Check that resuscitation equipment is readily available.

Indications for CS:

- status epilepticus
- uncontrolled repeated seizures
- fetal distress.

Management of fits in labour

- Call for help.
- Place woman in wedged position (to avoid vena cava compression).
- Keep head lower than the body, to allow any vomit to drain.
- Clear airways.
- Administer oxygen by facemask.
- Give IV lorazepam 4 mg bolus. If required, a further 1 mg bolus is given slowly. Use a large vein.
- Alternatively, IV diazepam 10 mg; further 2-mg boluses may be given if required, but do not exceed a total of 20 mg. If this fails to control seizures (ie status epilepticus), give IV phenytoin 15 mg/kg at an infusion rate ≤50 mg/minute.
- In status epilepticus, endotracheal intubation may be required.

Do not:

- leave the woman unattended
- restrain her
- put anything in her mouth
- give her anything by mouth until certain she is fully recovered.

After seizure:

■ Reassure woman when she recovers.
■ Make her comfortable (she may have had involuntary loss of urine during seizure).
■ CTG.

After delivery

Mother needs sleep, to reduce risk of seizure

Vitamin K 1 mg given to the baby at birth if the mother has been using anticonvulsant medication.

Encourage breastfeeding. Anticonvulsant drugs are excreted in breast milk in low concentrations but risks to the baby (irritability, lethargy) are minor compared with the benefits of breastfeeding. However, if the mother is on lamotrigine, warn that the baby may have a skin rash, in which case breastfeeding will have to be discontinued.

 Caution – fits could occur in the immediate postnatal period, resulting in accidents to mother and baby.

Advise regarding infant care to minimize danger to the baby in the event of the mother having a fit. Accidents could also occur during a bath or shower, so a midwife or health worker should be aware and the door should not be locked.

Review anticonvulsant medication and discuss contraception.

With the woman's consent, report to the UK Epilepsy and Pregnancy Register, Room 105, Bostock House, Royal Victoria Hospital, Grosvenor Road, Belfast BT12 6BA. Tel: (free-of-charge) 0800 389 1248.

Systemic lupus erythematosus

Principles

This is an immunological disorder in which antibodies are formed against own DNA and other cellular components. It is characterized by vasculitis and antinuclear antibodies. Other manifestations include cutaneous and neurological signs. The woman may present on the delivery suite with intrauterine fetal demise, pre-eclampsia, intrauterine growth restriction or preterm labour.

- Implement plan agreed and documented antenatally.
- Watch for
  - acute exacerbation in labour
  - hypertension
  - thrombosis
  - congenital heart block
  - neonatal lupus.
- Features of a flare include fever, arthralgia, myalgia, rash, oral ulcers, hypertension.

It may be difficult to distinguish lupus flare from pre-eclampsia. Also, pre-eclampsia may coexist with lupus flare. In lupus flare, urine microscopy shows red blood cells, leucocytes and granular casts.

- Transfer of antibodies across the placenta may result in congenital heart block.
- Paediatrician to be present at delivery.
- Caesarean section performed for obstetric indications.

Take the following action

☐ Continuous electronic fetal monitoring.
☐ Check full blood count, serum urate, creatinine, urea and electrolytes on admission.
☐ Urinalysis.
☐ Monitor hourly urine output.
☐ Alert anaesthetist.
☐ Alert paediatrician.
☐ Liaise with rheumatologist and immunology laboratory
☐ If on long-term steroid therapy, give hydrocortisone 100 mg IV every eight hours (three doses) because of inhibition of the pituitary–adrenal axis.
☐ If acute exacerbation occurs, discuss management with medical team. Steroids may be required.

Neonatal lupus:

Syndrome comprising congenital heart block, transient cutaneous lupus lesions and systemic manifestations. Occurs in 5% of babies born to women with systemic lupus erythematosus.

Other connective tissue disorders

 If on long-term steroid therapy, give hydrocortisone 100 mg IV every eight hours (three doses) because of inhibition of the pituitary–adrenal axis.

Rheumatoid arthritis

- If woman has been on nonsteroidal anti-inflammatory drugs (NSAIDs), watch for peripartum haemorrhage.
- Watch for pre-eclampsia.
- If woman is unable to fully abduct the hip, this may impede vaginal delivery.
- Rarely, atlanto-axial subluxation complicates general anaesthetic.
- Continuous electronic fetal monitoring.

Marfan syndrome

- Continuous electronic fetal monitoring.
- Check notes for plan agreed with cardiologist.
- If aortic root diameter >4 cm, recommend elective caesarean section (because of the risk of aortic dissection).
- Vaginal delivery in uncomplicated cases.
- If woman has heart-valve incompetence, give prophylactic antibiotics (see p. 177).

Ehlers–Danlos syndrome, types I–IX

These are inherited disorders of collagen metabolism, characterized by fragile skin and blood vessels, and hypermobility of the joints.

Types I and IV are more likely to develop complications in pregnancy, with a mortality rate of 20–25% in type IV disease. Prelabour rupture of membranes occurs frequently.

Malpresentation in labour is common, and the baby may be growth-restricted.

Potential problems include rupture of the great vessels during labour, vaginal and perineal tears, rupture of scar in women with previous caesarean section, difficulties with intubation, PPH, delayed wound healing and genital prolapse.

Mode of delivery to be decided by the consultant in discussion with the woman.

Part III: Haemorrhage and haematological disorders

6

The Rhesus-negative woman

Approximately 60% of babies born to Rhesus (D)-negative women in the UK are Rhesus-positive. Sensitized Rhesus-negative women with a significant antibody titre will usually be transferred to a tertiary centre. The following applies to non-sensitized women.

Following any potentially sensitizing event, such as trauma, placental abruption, vaginal bleeding, external cephalic version, amniocentesis:

- Give anti-D immunoglobulin 500–1000 units.
- Carry out Kleihauer test, then give additional anti-D if indicated.

At delivery

- Midwife who conducts delivery or receives the baby in theatre should obtain cord and maternal blood within two hours of delivery for a Kleihauer screening test.
- If unable to obtain cord blood, the midwife must perform a heel prick before the mother and baby are transferred to the postnatal ward.

All Rhesus-negative women who have given birth to a Rhesus-positive baby should be given anti-D within 72 hours of delivery.

If a Rhesus-negative woman receives platelet transfusion, check the product to confirm whether it is Rhesus-positive or Rhesus-negative platelet. If Rhesus-positive, then anti-D should be given (discuss with haematologist).

If a Rhesus-negative woman receives Rhesus-positive blood in error, discontinue transfusion immediately. Send maternal blood specimen for estimation of the volume of Rhesus-positive cells in circulation. Give anti-D 500 units for every 4 ml of Rhesus-positive blood transfused. Refer to local protocol for managing transfusion errors.

Thromboembolism prophylaxis

All women, irrespective of history, should have general measures (mobilization and avoidance of dehydration) to minimize the risk of venous thromboembolism.

Specific thromboprophylaxis is indicated in:

- all patients undergoing caesarean section
- women in normal labour and with a history of thrombosis, thrombophilia or other risk factors.

Thromboprophylaxis for caesarean section

All women undergoing caesarean section should be assessed for thromboembolism prophylaxis and given appropriate prophylaxis, depending on their risk category. A thromboembolism risk assessment form should be completed by the doctor obtaining consent for surgery.

Low risk

- elective caesarean section
- uncomplicated pregnancy and no other risk factors.

Prophylaxis:

☐ Thromboembolism-deterrent stockings (appropriate size and fitted correctly).
☐ Early mobilization and hydration.

Moderate risk

Woman with any one of the following risk factors:

- age >35 years
- obesity (>80 kg)
- ≥ para 4
- gross varicose veins
- current infection
- pre-eclampsia
- immobility before surgery (>4 days)
- major current illness, eg heart or lung disease, cancer, inflammatory bowel disease, nephrotic syndrome, sickle cell disease
- emergency caesarean section in labour
- excessive blood loss.

Prophylaxis:

☐ Thromboembolism-deterrent stockings or intermittent pneumatic compression.
☐ Early mobilization and hydration.
☐ Dalteparin (Fragmin) 5000 units SC daily until discharge.

High risk

- Two or more risk factors from the above.
- Extended major pelvic or abdominal surgery, eg caesarean, hysterectomy.
- Personal or family history of deep vein thrombosis, pulmonary embolism or thrombophilia.
- Paralysis of lower limbs.
- Antiphospholipid antibody (cardiolipin antibody or lupus anticoagulant).

Prophylaxis:

☐ Thromboembolism-deterrent stockings or pneumatic compression.
☐ Early mobilization and hydration.
☐ Dalteparin (Fragmin) 5000 units SC daily until the fifth postoperative day, or until fully ambulant if longer.
☐ Continue with dalteparin or warfarin for six weeks post-delivery.

The first dose of dalteparin should be given when the patient returns to the postnatal ward.

Thromboprophylaxis in vaginal deliveries

Many women requiring intrapartum thromboprophylaxis will have been identified antenatally. Some will have been commenced on heparin or aspirin earlier in pregnancy. Check notes for regime prescribed. For others, assess the risk and institute prophylaxis as follows.

Low risk

- Uncomplicated pregnancy.

Prophylaxis: Early mobilization and hydration.

Moderate risk

Woman with any two of the following risk factors:

- age >35 years
- obesity (>80 kg at booking)
- parity ≥4
- gross varicose veins
- current infection
- pre-eclampsia
- immobility before delivery (>4 days)

- major current illness, eg heart or lung disease, cancer, inflammatory bowel disease, nephrotic syndrome, sickle cell disease
- labour ≥12 hours
- excessive blood loss.

Prophylaxis:

☐ Early mobilization and hydration.
☐ Thromboembolism-deterrent stockings or pneumatic compression.
☐ Dalteparin 5000 units SC daily until discharge.

High risk

- Three or more risk factors from the above.
- Extended major pelvic or abdominal surgery, eg caesarean, hysterectomy.
- Personal or family history of deep vein thrombosis, pulmonary embolism or thrombophilia.
- paralysis of lower limbs.
- Antiphospholipid antibody (cardiolipin antibody or lupus anticoagulant).

Prophylaxis:

☐ Thromboembolism-deterrent stockings or pneumatic compression.
☐ Early mobilization and hydration.
☐ Dalteparin 5000 units SC daily until the fifth postoperative day, or until fully ambulant if longer.
☐ Continue with dalteparin or warfarin for six weeks post-delivery.

Dalteparin injection should be commenced within six hours of delivery.

Discuss with anaesthetist if epidural/spinal analgesia is planned (see also below). Thrombin time should be checked before the administration of an epidural/spinal block.

 Regional analgesia reduces the risk of DVT; general anaesthesia increases the risk of DVT.

 Thromboembolism-deterrent stockings could be harmful if fitted incorrectly.

Regional analgesia and dalteparin

Insertion of spinal/epidural block: at least 12 hours after last dose (this would apply mostly to women who have had antenatal prophylaxis).

Removal of epidural catheter: 12 hours after last dose.

After removal of catheter, wait at least six hours before administering next dose of dalteparin.

Acute venous thromboembolism and pulmonary embolism

Risk factors

- Obesity.
- Immobility.
- Grandmultiparity.
- Previous deep vein thrombosis.
- Dehydration.
- Surgical procedures.
- Antepartum or postpartum haemorrhage.
- Pre-eclampsia.
- Thrombophilia (see p 158).
- Age >35 years.
- Infection.
- Operative delivery.
- Sickle cell disease.
- Inflammatory disorder.
- Long-distance travel.

Clinical features

- Leg pain, swelling or tenderness.
- Chest pain, breathlessness, haemoptysis.
- Faintness, collapse.
- Pyrexia.
- Raised jugular venous pressure.

Initial investigation

☐ Full blood count.
☐ Urea and electrolytes, liver function tests.
☐ Coagulation screen.
☐ D-dimer (green-top bottle).
☐ Thrombophilia screen (if starting on anticoagulant; see below).

Suspected DVT:

☐ Compression or duplex ultrasound scan.

Suspected PE:

☐ Pulse oximetry.

☐ Arterial blood gases.
☐ ECG.
☐ Chest X-ray.
☐ Ventilation–perfusion scan.
☐ Doppler ultrasound leg studies (bilateral).

Any woman with signs or symptoms suggestive of VTE should undergo diagnostic imaging to confirm or exclude the diagnosis.

 The D-dimer test is a negative predictive test: a low level suggests there is no VTE but a high level may be normal in pregnancy.

If it is not possible to perform diagnostic imaging on the same day, then treatment should be initiated whilst awaiting objective diagnosis, *unless treatment is strongly contraindicated.*

If ultrasound scan for DVT is negative but clinical suspicion is high, then continue anticoagulant treatment and request a venogram.

Management

- See algorithms, Figures 6 and 7, pp. 150–151.
- Consult haematologist.
- Graduated elastic compression stockings.
- Anticoagulant treatment (see below).
- Deep vein thrombosis: measure leg circumference daily.
- Encourage ambulation.

Anticoagulant therapy for deep vein thrombosis and pulmonary embolism

The woman should be screened for thrombophilia before anticoagulant therapy is commenced.

Thrombophilia screen (two EDTA bottles plus three citrate bottles; indicate on card the gestational age):

- anticardiolipin antibodies
- lupus anticoagulant
- protein C
- protein S
- activated protein C resistance
- factor V Leiden mutation
- prothrombin G20210A mutation.

As levels of some of these factors vary in pregnancy, the results should be interpreted in consultation with the haematologist.

Low-molecular-weight heparin

Low-molecular-weight heparin (LMWH) is the anticoagulant of choice, barring any special considerations (see next page for special circumstances).

Dose is weight-related. Use the weight at booking or current weight minus 10%.

 To work out the dose required: dalteparin 100 units/kg SC twice daily.

Prescribe and use prefilled syringe (from a choice of 2500, 5000, 10 000 and 12 500 units) nearest to the calculated requirement.

Do not use less than 10 000 units or more than 18 000 units in 24 hours.

Measure peak anti-Xa level three hours post-injection, aiming for a therapeutic range of 0.5–1 units/ml. Adjust level of dalteparin as advised by haematologist, reassessing anti-Xa activity after each dose adjustment.

Check platelet count on days two and seven after commencement of dalteparin.

Intravenous unfractionated heparin

This has a shorter half-life than LMWH and is readily reversible with protamine sulphate, so should be used in the following circumstances:

- massive pulmonary embolism
- floating thrombus on ultrasound scan
- prosthetic valve
- renal failure
- increased risk of bleeding (eg as result of coagulopathy, trauma, surgery, peptic ulcer)
- wound haematoma
- antepartum or postpartum haemorrhage.

Ensure baseline clotting and platelet count are normal before starting.

Loading dose: 5000 units IV over 5 minutes.

Maintenance infusion: use a preparation of 1000 units /ml. Start at 1 ml/hour (ie 1000 units/hour).

Check activated partial thromboplastin time (APTT) four to six hours after loading dose, aiming for a therapeutic target of 2–2.5 times the average laboratory control value.

Adjust infusion rate as advised by haematologist, and recheck APTT every four to six hours until the therapeutic ratio is reached. Once the therapeutic ratio is reached, check APTT at least daily.

In some pregnancies, the therapeutic ratio is difficult to achieve despite high doses of heparin, because fibrinogen and factor VIII levels rise in pregnancy. In such cases, anti-Xa activity should be monitored, aiming for a range of 0.35–0.70 units /ml.

Check platelet count on days two, seven and ten.

Contraindications to heparin (including LMWH)

- Active bleeding.
- Where surgical treatment is to be undertaken, eg caval filter, embolectomy.
- Previous heparin-induced thrombocytopenia (use danaparoid).
- Previous heparin skin allergy (discuss with haematologist).

Duration of treatment

Following treatment of the acute phase, anticoagulation should be maintained with LMWH for at least six months. In many cases, it would be safe to reduce anticoagulation to a prophylactic dose. Arrange follow-up appointment with the haematology/coagulation clinic.

Labour and delivery

A woman on therapeutic anticoagulation should be delivered by planned induction of labour or elective CS at 37–38 weeks. She should be advised that in the event of contractions starting before the day of admission, no further heparin should be self-administered until she has been assessed in hospital.

Women on prophylactic dose may await spontaneous onset of labour.

Induction of labour

- [ ] Omit evening dose of dalteparin before admission.
- [ ] On admission: full blood count, coagulation profile, anti-Xa, group-and-save.
- [ ] Inform haematologist.
- [ ] Dalteparin 5000 units daily (ie prophylactic dose) given on admission and continued until delivered.
- [ ] Thromboembolism-deterrent stockings.
- [ ] Active management of third stage.
- [ ] Syntocinon infusion 40 units in 500 ml Hartmann's solution or normal saline for four hours post-delivery.
- [ ] Therapeutic regime resumed following delivery.

Elective caesarean section

- [ ] Omit evening dose before day of operation.
- [ ] On admission: full blood count, coagulation profile, anti-Xa, group-and-save.
- [ ] Inform haematologist.

☐ Give dalteparin 5000 units SC three hours postoperative, or four hours after removal of epidural catheter.

☐ Consider placing a wound drain.

☐ Use staples or interrupted sutures for skin.

☐ Syntocinon infusion 40 units in 500 ml Hartmann's solution or normal saline for four hours post-delivery.

☐ Therapeutic regime resumed the evening after surgery.

☐ Thromboembolism-deterrent stockings.

Epidural or spinal anaesthesia

This should be discussed with the woman before induction of labour or CS.

If the woman is on a therapeutic dose of LMWH, then regional block should not be used until at least 24 hours after the last dose.

If the woman is on a prophylactic dose (this should be the case if the above protocol for induction and elective CS has been followed), then regional block should not be used until at least 12 hours after the last dose.

LMWH should not be given for at least six hours after the epidural catheter has been removed. The cannula should not be removed within 12 hours of the most recent injection.

Postpartum anticoagulation

Anticoagulation should be continued for at least six weeks. If the woman opts for oral anticoagulant (warfarin), this can be started on the day following delivery. Breastfeeding is not a contraindication to warfarin.

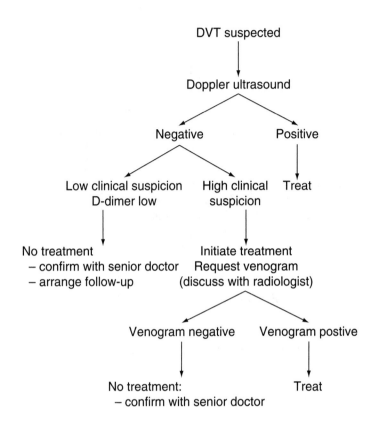

Figure 6   *Algorithm for suspected DVT*

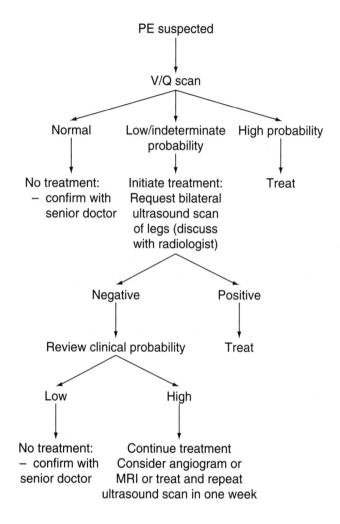

Figure 7 *Algorithm for suspected PE*

Major haemoglobinopathy

Major haemoglobinopathies are sickle cell disease and thalassaemia. These should be excluded in women of African, Asian or Mediterranean origin. In particular, major haemoglobinopathy should be suspected when there is anaemia in the absence of bleeding in any of these populations (but haemoglobinopathy is not exclusive to these). A sickle cell crisis may be precipitated or exacerbated by hypoxia/acidosis, dehydration and infection.

Principles of management in labour

- Avoid dehydration, infection, acidosis, hypoxia and prolonged labour.
- Liaise with haematologist and blood transfusion laboratory.
- Inform anaesthetist and paediatrician on admission.
- If administering Syntocinon drip, avoid fluid overload.
- In cases of prelabour rupture of membranes, labour should be induced to minimize the risk of chorioamnionitis.
- Do not give iron supplement.

Action plan

- [ ] Record blood pressure and urinalysis on admission.
- [ ] Check full blood count, urea and electrolytes, liver function tests, urates, creatinine and blood gases on admission.
- [ ] Establish IV access.
- [ ] Cross-match four units of blood.
- [ ] Continuous CTG monitoring.
- [ ] Pulse oximetry.
- [ ] Oxygen.
- [ ] Liberal oral fluid intake or judicious use of IV fluids.
- [ ] Antibiotic cover – penicillin.
- [ ] Recommend epidural analgesia, especially where operative delivery is anticipated, but:
  - avoid overload when giving IV fluid before epidural
  - use elastic stockings and leg elevation to avoid hypotension and venous pooling in legs.
- [ ] Watch for signs of pulmonary embolism.
- [ ] Consider thromboembolism prophylaxis.
- [ ] Active management of third stage.
- [ ] Take cord blood for full blood count and haemoglobin electrophoresis.

Sickle cell crisis

Bone pain crisis: fever, painful limbs, chest and abdomen, tender bones and abdomen.

Sequestration: bone pain, abdominal pain, fever, hepatomegaly, splenomegaly, falling [Hb].

Aplastic crisis: fever, dyspnoea, pallor, low [Hb], low reticulocyte count.

☐ Involve haematologist.
☐ Maintain airway oxygen via face mask 15 l/min.
☐ Assess pulse and blood pressure.
☐ Monitor O_2 saturation.
☐ ECG.
☐ IV access, full blood count, urea and electrolytes, reticulocyte count, liver function tests.
☐ Arterial blood gases.
☐ Sepsis screen: blood culture, mid-stream specimen of urine for bacteriology.
☐ Chest X-ray if there are chest symptoms.
☐ Rehydrate with Hartmann's solution or normal saline.
☐ Monitor fluid input and urine output.
☐ Parenteral analgesia.
☐ IV antibiotics.
☐ Treat cause of crisis if identified.
☐ Cross-match four units of blood (laboratory must be informed that woman has sickle cell disease).
☐ Transfusion as required (packed cells) – discuss with haematologist. Not usually required if [Hb] ≥6 g/dl.

Inherited coagulation disorders: haemophilia and von Willebrand disease

Coagulation disorders can be inherited or acquired:

- *Inherited:* haemophilia, von Willebrand disease, factor XI deficiency and other rare disorders.
- *Acquired:* gestational thrombocytopoenia, immune thrombocytopenic purpura (ITP, p. 156).

Haemophilia

Haemophilia A is due to deficiency of factor VIII. Haemophilia B is due to deficiency of factor IX. Both are X-linked recessive disorders. Most carriers do not have bleeding problems, but a small number have a tendency to bleed, due to low clotting factor levels that result from lyonization or homozygosity.

Von Willebrand disease

A group of autosomally inherited disorders. Von Willebrand factor (vWF) is essential for normal platelet function and acts as a carrier for factor VIII, so patients with this disease usually have prolonged bleeding time and reduced factor VIIIc activity.

Classified into three types: in types 1 and 3, there is reduced synthesis of von Willebrand factor (vWF), but the structure is normal; in type 2, the amount of factor produced may be normal, but the structure is abnormal. Bleeding is more frequent and more severe in types 2 and 3.

The incidence of primary PPH is high, and the incidence of secondary PPH is even higher. Secondary PPH may be treated with tranexamic acid. In severe cases, discuss with haematologist regarding treatment with DDAVP (desmopressin acetate) or vWF concentrate.

Action plan

☐ Check notes for plan agreed with consultant haematologist.
☐ Ascertain availability of blood product as required (see below).
☐ Full blood count.
☐ Coagulation tests.
☐ Check clotting factor levels (factor VIIIc in haemophilia A, factor IXc in haemophilia B).
☐ Group-and-save.

☐ Avoid intramuscular injections.

☐ Epidural analgesia may be given provided that coagulation screen is normal and platelet count is >100×10⁹/l. Epidural is also considered safe if coagulation factor levels are >50 IU/dl.

☐ Repeat coagulation screen before removing epidural catheter.

☐ Avoid use of fetal scalp electrode and fetal scalp blood sampling, as an affected fetus may bleed.

☐ Early recourse to caesarean section in cases of slow progress.

☐ Avoid ventouse delivery (low forceps may be performed and is preferable to a traumatic caesarean section delivery).

☐ If caesarean section or instrumental delivery required, ensure clotting factor levels are >50 IU/l. If clotting factor level <50 IU/l, transfuse with recombinant factor VIII or IX, as appropriate.

☐ Anticipate postpartum haemorrhage (PPH).

☐ Obtain cord blood for investigation.

☐ Give neonate oral vitamin K.

☐ Post-delivery, ensure that clotting factor activity is >50 IU/dl for five days, to minimize risk of PPH.

☐ Inform GP so that the neonate's immunizations are given subcutaneously or intradermally.

Immune thrombocytopenic purpura

Immune thrombocytopenic purpura (ITP) is a condition in which platelets are destroyed prematurely by antiplatelet antibodies. There is no diagnostic test; the condition is diagnosed by exclusion of other causes of thrombocytopenia. The platelet count is persistently low (<100×10⁹/l), but the FBC, blood film, PT and APTT are normal. Tests for antiplatelet antibodies are non-specific and do not distinguish ITP from gestational thrombocytopenia. Bone-marrow biopsy may be needed for diagnosis.

When seen on the delivery suite, the woman will fall into one of the following groups, depending on what treatment she has received:

- *Asymptomatic and with platelet count >50×10⁹/l:* requires no treatment.
- *Been on prednisolone for maintenance of platelet count:* give hydrocortisone 100 mg IV every eight hours to cover labour and delivery (because of inhibition of the pituitary–adrenal axis).
- *IV immunoglobulin given just before induction of labour or caesarean section:* watch for side-effects of headache, nausea, alopecia and abnormal liver function tests.

Action plan

- ☐ Check notes for plan agreed with consultant haematologist.
- ☐ Full blood count.
- ☐ Liver function tests.
- ☐ Coagulation profile.
- ☐ Check clotting factor levels.
- ☐ Confirm availability and access to platelets for transfusion.
- ☐ Alert paediatricians (the baby is at risk of thrombocytopenia, which carries a risk of intracranial haemorrhage).
- ☐ Avoid intramuscular injection of pethidine.
- ☐ Discuss pain relief with consultant anaesthetist.
- ☐ Epidural not contraindicated if:
  - full blood count normal
  - coagulation profile normal
  - clotting factor levels >50 IU/l during third trimester.
- ☐ Check factor levels before removing epidural catheter.
- ☐ Obtain anticoagulated cord blood sample and send immediately to haemophilia laboratory.

Mode of delivery

Mode of delivery remains controversial. In each case, it should be decided by the consultant obstetrician and consultant haematologist, with the consent of the woman. If platelet count $<50\times10^9/l$, then platelet transfusion and CS may decrease the risk of intracranial haemorrhage in the neonate.

Avoid the use of fetal scalp electrode and ventouse delivery.

The neonate

Antiplatelet antibodies may cross the placenta, causing fetal thrombocytopenia. This may manifest as purpura, haematuria or intracranial haemorrhage. Neither prednisolone therapy nor intravenous immunoglobulin given to the mother can prevent fetal thrombocytopenia.

The risk of bleeding is low if the fetus has a platelet count $>50\times10^9/l$, but obtaining a sample of fetal blood is risky and requires special skills.

Action:

- Give vitamin K orally.
- Routine immunizations should be given subcutaneously or intradermally.
- Consider hepatitis B immunization.

Thrombophilia

Thrombophilia is an abnormality of haemostasis predisposing to thrombosis. It may be:

- *hereditary:*
  - activated protein C resistance (associated with factor V Leiden mutation)
  - protein C deficiency
  - protein S deficiency
  - antithrombin deficiency
  - prothrombin gene mutation
- *acquired:*
  - antiphospholipid syndrome
  - polycythaemia
  - other conditions such as malignancy.

Hyperhomocysteinaemia is a thrombophilia with genetic and acquired origins.

About 50% of thromboembolic events in pregnancy occur in women with an identifiable thrombophilia.

Women with thrombophilia are also at increased risk of stillbirth, intrauterine growth restriction and pre-eclampsia.

Management in labour

Most women with known thrombophilia will have been commenced on anticoagulant treatment antenatally.

☐ Check notes for management plan as outlined by consultant obstetrician/ haematologist.
☐ Discontinue heparin/dalteparin if in labour or before induction of labour.
☐ Full blood count.
☐ Coagulation screen: activated partial thromboplastin time (APTT), prothrombin time (PT), anti-Xa assay (if available).
☐ Watch for pre-eclampsia developing in labour.

Epidural analgesia may be considered if:

- heparin/dalteparin has not been given in the preceding six hours
- coagulation screen is normal
- platelet count is >100×10^9/l.

Postpartum

- Resume anticoagulant prophylaxis 12 hours after delivery (unless bleeding in excess of lochial loss).
- Continue anticoagulant prophylaxis for three months.
- May start oral anticoagulants within the first two days, and withdraw heparin/dalteparin when International Normalized Ratio (INR) has been within the therapeutic range for three days.
- In cases of heritable thrombophilia, inform parents of risk of autosomal transmission.

Gestational thrombocytopenia

Mild reduction in platelet count occurring in the second or third trimester, with no bleeding problems to mother and baby. The platelet count is usually 100–150×10^9/l and reverts to normal after pregnancy.

Vaginal delivery is safe.

Regional analgesia is safe.

Antepartum haemorrhage

Defined formally as bleeding from the genital tract after 24 weeks' gestation. In practice, vaginal bleeding that occurs after a woman has had a normal fetal anatomy scan is managed as antepartum haemorrhage (APH).

Differential diagnosis

- placenta praevia (see p. 164)
- placental abruption (concealed bleeding could be more significant than revealed loss)
- bleeding from the cervix (ectopy, polyp, carcinoma, etc)
- vasa praevia.

Assessment

☐ Assess blood loss.
☐ Check blood pressure, pulse and respiration.
☐ If in shock: airway, breathing, circulation.
☐ Exclude abdominal pain and contractions.
☐ Exclude placenta praevia before doing digital vaginal examination.

! Note that abruption of a posterior placenta may present as back pain.

Minor antepartum haemorrhage (minimal loss on admission)

☐ Check scan reports for placental site (but note that scans can be wrong).
☐ Speculum examination.
☐ Full blood count, group-and-save, Kleihauer if Rhesus-negative.
☐ CTG.
☐ If Rhesus-negative, give anti-D 1000 units IM.
☐ Transfer to ward if no major bleeding, uterine tenderness or fetal distress.

Moderate antepartum haemorrhage (significant bleeding but not in shock)

☐ IV line (14G).
☐ Full blood count, urea and electrolytes, clotting, cross-match four units, Kleihauer if Rhesus-negative.

- [ ] Catheterize and monitor urine output.
- [ ] Intensive monitoring chart.
- [ ] Inform anaesthetist and neonatal unit.
- [ ] Inform consultant: decision to be made regarding mode and timing of delivery.
- [ ] If Rhesus-negative and delivery not imminent, give anti-D 1000 units IM.
- [ ] Monitor on delivery suite for at least 12 hours post-delivery.

Major antepartum haemorrhage (estimated loss >1000 ml)

- [ ] Call for senior obstetrician, anaesthetist, theatre team and porters. Alert blood bank and haematology laboratory.
- [ ] Oxygen by mask – 8 l/min.
- [ ] Keep the woman warm.
- [ ] Two IV lines with 14G, or larger, cannula.
- [ ] Catheterize and monitor urine output.
- [ ] ECG.
- [ ] Pulse oximetry.
- [ ] Serial blood pressure recording.
- [ ] Consider central venous pressure monitoring and arterial line.

This is likely to be required if blood loss in excess of 1500 ml or if the woman is to be taken to theatre.

> **!** 'Failure to use [CVP] monitoring in the treatment of major obstetric haemorrhage is substandard care' – Thomas TA, Cooper GM. Anaesthesia. In: Lewis G (ed). *Why Mothers Die 1997–99, The Confidential Enquiries into Maternal Deaths in the United Kingdom*. London: RCOG Press, 2001, p. 143.

- [ ] Full blood count, prothrombin time (PT), activated partial thrombopastin time (APTT), fibrin degradation products (FDP) and fibrinogen.
- [ ] Urgent cross-match six units of blood.
- [ ] Give plasma substitutes: Haemaccel or Gelofusine 1000 ml immediately.
- [ ] Transfuse cross-matched blood if available
- [ ] If cross-matched blood not available immediately, use:
  - unmatched blood (patient's group) usually available within 15 minutes
  - group 0 negative blood (emergency stock) – if blood needed immediately.
- [ ] *Before using uncross-matched blood, always:*
  - *discuss with laboratory*
  - *obtain the woman's blood sample for tests listed above.*
- [ ] Use one unit fresh-frozen plasma for every eight units of packed cells. Further transfusion of coagulation factors may be required – see 'Transfusion of clotting factors'.

> **!** Blood-warming equipment should be used.

☐ Continuous CTG monitoring.
☐ Record blood loss: weigh soaked linen.
☐ If CTG normal and bleeding has settled, ultrasound scan. Scan also indicated if fetal heart tones not detected.

Transfusion of clotting factors

The clinical situation may have changed by the time blood results are available, so treat the patient not the results. Treat coagulation defects as advised by haematologist. Transfusion of fresh frozen plasma (FFP) is usually required if blood loss/replacement approaches the estimated blood volume of the woman. Platelet transfusion is usually needed with 1.5–2 times blood volume replacement. Cryoprecipitate is likely to be needed if fibrinogen level is abnormally low.

> 'A standing agreement between the haematologists and obstetricians over the issue of platelets, FFP and cryoprecipitate reduces the number of phone calls required and speeds response. Coagulation monitoring will help to assess the adequacy of the coagulation support and guide the selection of components but should not delay the initial issue of FFP or cryoprecipitate.'
>
> – Blood Transfusion Services of the United Kingdom. Obstetric Haemorrhage. In: McClelland DBL (ed). *Handbook of Transfusion Medicine*, 3rd edn. London: The Stationery Office, 2001, p. 80

Senior obstetrician makes the decision regarding urgency and mode of delivery.

Consider early transfer to ITU/HDU.

Delivery

Active management of third stage of labour.

APH predisposes to PPH, so a Syntocinon infusion (40 units in 500 ml Hartmann's solution or normal saline) should be commenced in the third stage of labour and continued for four hours post-delivery.

Major placenta praevia

Vaginal delivery is contraindicated if the placenta encroaches within 2 cm of the internal os.

Elective or emergency caesarean section for major placenta praevia should be performed only by a consultant obstetrician or by an experienced obstetrician with the consultant in attendance.

Action plan

☐ Discuss possibility of blood transfusion.
☐ Cross-match four to six units of blood.
☐ In cases of anterior placenta praevia in a scarred uterus (ie previous caesarean section), the woman should be informed of the possibility of placenta accreta. Consent should be obtained for a hysterectomy to be performed in the event of uncontrollable bleeding.
☐ Anticipate postpartum haemorrhage: commence Syntocinon infusion (40 units in 500 ml Hartmann's solution or normal saline) immediately after delivery of the baby.

 In the event of massive haemorrhage, manage as outlined on pp. 162–163.

Retained placenta

Definition: placenta has shown no signs of separation after 20 minutes of delivery of the baby (60 minutes if the third stage has been managed physiologically).

The plan below also applies when the placenta has been delivered but there are missing cotyledons.

 In cases of a scarred uterus, beware of placenta accreta. Obtain consent for possible blood transfusion and hysterectomy before proceeding to manual removal.

In some cases of retained placenta, the placenta will separate following injection of a mixture of Syntocinon 10–20 units and 20 ml normal saline into the umbilical vein.

Action plan

☐ Inform registrar.
☐ Ensure bladder is empty.
☐ IV line (14G or larger).
☐ Syntocinon infusion 40 units in 500 ml Hartmann's solution or normal saline.
☐ Group-and-save (cross-match if bleeding more than 500 ml).
☐ Monitor pulse, blood pressure and blood loss.
☐ Counsel regarding possibility of placenta accreta.
☐ Manual removal of retained placenta in theatre under spinal or epidural analgesia. (General anaesthetic preferable only if patient is shocked or bleeding heavily.)
☐ If placenta is morbidly adherent, call consultant immediately.
☐ Continue Syntocinon infusion for four. hours after manual removal.
☐ IV co-amoxiclav (Augmentin) or cefuroxime/metronidazole given as bolus.
☐ If uterine inversion occurs in the process of manual removal, then reduce the inversion before any further attempt at removing the placenta. Call consultant immediately. See also p. 196.

Postpartum haemorrhage

! Only two-thirds of all PPHs occur in women with known risk factors.

! At CS, blood loss is likely to be higher if the placenta is removed manually than if it were removed by cord traction.

Action plan

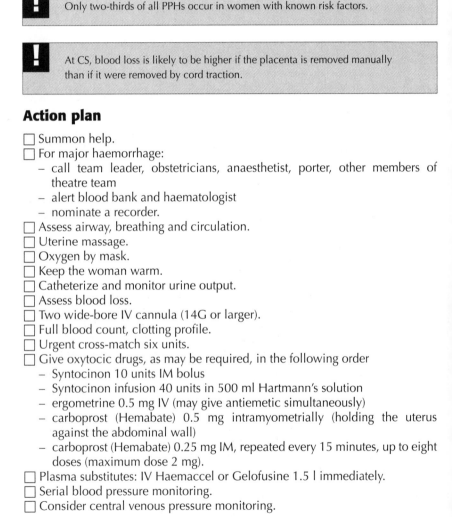

- [ ] Summon help.
- [ ] For major haemorrhage:
  - call team leader, obstetricians, anaesthetist, porter, other members of theatre team
  - alert blood bank and haematologist
  - nominate a recorder.
- [ ] Assess airway, breathing and circulation.
- [ ] Uterine massage.
- [ ] Oxygen by mask.
- [ ] Keep the woman warm.
- [ ] Catheterize and monitor urine output.
- [ ] Assess blood loss.
- [ ] Two wide-bore IV cannula (14G or larger).
- [ ] Full blood count, clotting profile.
- [ ] Urgent cross-match six units.
- [ ] Give oxytocic drugs, as may be required, in the following order
  - Syntocinon 10 units IM bolus
  - Syntocinon infusion 40 units in 500 ml Hartmann's solution
  - ergometrine 0.5 mg IV (may give antiemetic simultaneously)
  - carboprost (Hemabate) 0.5 mg intramyometrially (holding the uterus against the abdominal wall)
  - carboprost (Hemabate) 0.25 mg IM, repeated every 15 minutes, up to eight doses (maximum dose 2 mg).
- [ ] Plasma substitutes: IV Haemaccel or Gelofusine 1.5 l immediately.
- [ ] Serial blood pressure monitoring.
- [ ] Consider central venous pressure monitoring.

'Failure to use [CVP] monitoring in the treatment of major obstetric haemorrhage is substandard care' – Thomas TA, Cooper GM. Anaesthesia. In: Lewis G (ed). *Why Mothers Die 1997–99. The Confidential Enquiries into Maternal Deaths in the United Kingdom.* London: RCOG Press, 2001, p. 143.

☐ Record pulse rate, blood pressure, oxygen saturation, central venous pressure and other observations on high-dependency chart.

☐ Diagnose and treat source of bleeding: the four Ts – tone, trauma, tissue (placenta), thrombin (clotting).

Retained placenta: proceed immediately to manual removal.

Uterine atony: oxytocic regime as above. May also consider use of Bakri or Sengstaken–Blakemore tube. Before using the tube, ensure there are no retained products of conception. Inflate balloon with 300 ml normal saline. Leave for 24 hours, then deflate at a rate of 20 ml/hour.

Genital tract trauma or undiagnosed bleeding: proceed to examination under anaesthetic (EUA). Counsel for laparotomy and possible hysterectomy. Good light and good assistance are essential for EUA.

Coagulopathy: Manage in collaboration with haematologist. The clinical situation may have changed by the time blood results are available, so treat the patient not the results. Treat coagulation defects as advised by haematologist. Transfusion of fresh frozen plasma (FFP) is usually required if blood loss/replacement approaches the estimated blood volume of the woman. Platelet transfusion is usually needed with 1.5–2 times blood volume replacement. Cryoprecipitate is likely to be needed if fibrinogen level is abnormally low.

'A standing agreement between the haematologists and obstetricians over the issue of platelets, FFP and cryoprecipitate reduces the number of phone calls required and speeds response. Coagulation monitoring will help to assess the adequacy of the coagulation support and guide the selection of components but should not delay the initial issue of FFP or cryoprecipitate.'

– Blood Transfusion Services of the United Kingdom. Obstetric Haemorrhage. In: McClelland DBL (ed). *Handbook of Transfusion Medicine,* 3rd edn. London: The Stationery Office, 2001, p. 80

☐ Frequency of repeat blood tests is determined by clinical situation but in major bleeding would usually be every four hours until stable.

☐ Estimate the blood loss – weigh soaked linen and swabs.

☐ Consider early transfer to HDU or ITU.

Take care: in the rush to get things done, a blood specimen is sometimes sent to the laboratory either unlabelled or with incorrect identity.

Blood transfusion

■ Transfuse cross-matched blood if available.
■ If cross-matched blood not available immediately, may use:
  – unmatched blood (patient's group) – usually available within 15 minutes
  – group 0 negative blood (emergency stock) – given if blood needed immediately, ie life-threatening situation.
■ *Before using uncross-matched blood, always:*
  – *discuss with laboratory*
  – *obtain the woman's blood sample for tests listed above.*
■ Use blood-warming equipment.
■ Infuse with a pressure bag.

Where do things usually go wrong?

■ Failure to anticipate high-risk patients.
■ Being falsely reassured by a systolic blood pressure above 100 mmHg. Usually systolic pressure does not fall until a minimum of 1.5 l has been lost.
■ Inadequate blood transfusion or excessive use of fluids.
■ Failure to detect early disseminated intravascular coagulation (DIC).
■ Lack of involvement of senior staff at an early stage.
■ Delay in resort to surgical treatment.

Disseminated intravascular coagulopathy

DIC should be anticipated in severe pre-eclampsia, APH, PPH, placental abruption, amniotic fluid embolism and septicaemia.

Early involvement of the haematologist is vital.

Investigations

☐ Full blood count.
☐ Group and cross-match four to six units of blood.
☐ Coagulation profile.

Low fibrinogen and elevated FDP levels are indicative of decompensation.

Treatment

- High-dependency care.
- Manage shock.
- Liaise with consultant haematologist (re: blood product support).
- Treat underlying cause.
- See protocol for management of massive haemorrhage (pp. 162–163).

Delivery of woman at known risk of haemorrhage

A higher risk of major bleeding at delivery should be anticipated in the following cases:

- previous PPH
- placenta praevia
- significant uterine fibroids
- previous myomectomy
- placental abruption
- multiple pregnancy
- antepartum haemorrhage
- significant uterine fibroids
- grandmultiparity
- retained placenta
- macrosomia
- prolonged labour.

Women at risk should have:

- 14FG IV cannula in labour
- full blood count, group-and-save on admission
- bladder emptied in third stage of labour
- active management of third stage of labour.

Syntocinon infusion 40 units in 500ml normal saline (or Hartmann's) for 4 hours after delivery.

Where surgery is indicated:

All elective and emergency surgery should be performed by a consultant or by an experienced obstetrician with a consultant in attendance.

Senior anaesthetist should be involved. Elective CS for placenta praevia and other potentially difficult cases should be scheduled for a session when a consultant anaesthetist is available.

☐ Place two 14FG IV cannulae before surgery.
☐ Cross-match four units of blood. These should be immediately available.
☐ Insert central venous pressure line (either preoperatively or when bleeding is excessive).

Liaise with consultant haematologist in cases of coagulopathy.

See also management of PPH, pp. 166–168, and management of major placenta praevia, p. 164.

Management of the woman who declines blood transfusion

Some women decline transfusion because of specific personal or religious beliefs. The main group of women who may refuse for religious reason are members of the Jehovah's Witnesses.

If it is thought likely that a woman may refuse blood transfusion, then management of massive haemorrhage should be considered in advance.

Booking

Discuss risks of withholding blood transfusion (in a non-confrontational, non-judgemental manner). The woman and her partner should be offered the opportunity to read and discuss the guidance given below.

She should be asked if she is willing to receive blood transfusion in a life-threatening emergency, and her reply should be noted. This reply, given without duress, constitutes an advance directive. She should sign the appropriate form indicating her refusal of blood or blood products.

Antenatal care

Blood group and antibody status: check at booking, 30 weeks and 36 weeks

Haemoglobin and serum ferritin: check at 36 weeks.

Haematinics should be given throughout pregnancy to maximize iron stores.

If ultrasound scan shows a low-lying placenta, then the implications should be discussed with the woman.

 Blood storage for autotransfusion should not be suggested to pregnant women as the amounts of blood required to treat massive obstetric haemorrhage are far in excess of the amount that could be donated during pregnancy.

The consultant obstetrician must be kept informed of any antenatal complications.

Labour

☐ On admission, inform consultant obstetrician and consultant anaesthetist.
☐ The third stage of labour should be managed actively.
☐ The woman should be observed closely for at least an hour after delivery.

If CS is necessary, it should be carried out by a consultant obstetrician if possible.

When the mother is discharged from hospital, she should be advised to report any bleeding promptly.

Management of haemorrhage

The principle is to avoid delay. Rapid decision-making may be necessary, particularly with regard to surgical intervention.

☐ Inform consultant obstetrician.
☐ Inform consultant anaesthetist.
☐ Inform consultant haematologist.
☐ Commence promptly standard management (short of blood transfusion) described for ante-/postnatal haemorrhage (see pp. 161–163 and 166–168).

The threshold for intervention should be lower than in other patients.

Extra vigilance should be exercised to quantify any abnormal bleeding and to detect complications, such as clotting abnormalities, as promptly as possible.

Communication

- Keep the woman fully informed about what is happening. Information must be given in a professional way, ideally by someone who the woman knows and trusts.
- Maintain a professional attitude. Do not lose the trust of the patient or her partner, since further decisions, eg regarding hysterectomy, may have to be made.
- If standard treatment is not controlling the bleeding, advise the woman that blood transfusion is strongly recommended. She is entitled to change her mind about a previously agreed treatment plan.
- Be satisfied that the woman is not being subjected to pressure from others. It is reasonable to ask the accompanying persons to leave the room for a while so that the doctor (with a midwife or other colleague) can ask the woman whether she is making her decision of her own free will.
- If the woman maintains her refusal to accept blood or blood products, then her wishes must be respected.

Drugs and infusions

Dextran should be avoided for fluid replacement because of its possible effects on haemostasis. Intravenous crystalloid and plasma substitutes (Haemaccel or Gelofusine) should be used. In cases of severe bleeding, IV vitamin K should be given to the woman. Other drugs that have been recommended include desmopressin, methylprednisolone and fibrinolytic inhibitors, such as aprotinin and tranexamic acid.

The advice of the haematologist should be sought before considering the use of heparin to combat disseminated intravascular coagulation.

If the woman survives the acute episode and is transferred to ITU, management there should include erythropoietin, parenteral iron therapy and adequate protein for haemoglobin synthesis.

Hysterectomy

Hysterectomy is usually a treatment of last resort in obstetric haemorrhage, but for a woman who declines blood transfusion any delay may increase the risk of death. The timing of hysterectomy is an on-the-spot decision for the consultant.

When hysterectomy is performed, the uterine arteries should be clamped as early as possible in the procedure. Subtotal hysterectomy can be just as effective as total hysterectomy, and is quicker and safer.

In some cases, there may be a place for ligation of the internal iliac artery.

 If, in spite of all care, the woman dies, then her relatives require support like any other bereaved family.

Management of staff

It is distressing for staff to have to watch a woman bleed to death while refusing effective treatment. Support should be available for staff in these circumstances.

Part IV: Infection

Prophylactic antibiotics

Caesarean section

All women undergoing elective or emergency CS should have a single-dose prophylactic antibiotic: IV cefuroxime 750 mg given after clamping of the cord.

If there are two or more of the following risk factors for postoperative wound infection, then consider giving a full course of antibiotics:

- prolonged rupture of membranes (>12 hours)
- prolonged labour (>8 hours)
- multiple vaginal examinations (>5 in the past 24 hours)
- obesity (body mass index >30 at booking).

Cardiac disease

All women in labour and with a structural heart defect, prosthetic valve or history of endocarditis must have prophylactic antibiotics:

- *Caesarean section:* amoxicillin 1 g IV and gentamicin 120 mg IV (over 3 minutes) at induction of anaesthesia, then amoxicillin 500 mg six hours later.
- *Vaginal delivery:* amoxicillin 1 g IV and gentamicin 120 mg IV (over 3 minutes) at onset of labour or ruptured membranes, then amoxicillin 500 mg six hours later.
- *Woman allergic to penicillin or who has had more than a single dose of penicillin in the previous month:* vancomycin 1 g by slow IV infusion (over at least 60 minutes) before delivery, then gentamicin 120 mg IV at induction of anaesthesia or at rupture of membranes.

Group B streptococci

See pp. 180–181.

Prolonged rupture of fetal membranes

Commence after 18 hours. Same regime as for group B streptococci (see pp. 180–181). See also prelabour rupture of membranes, p. 23.

Intrapartum pyrexia

Principles

- Look for focus of infection: respiratory, cardiac, urinary tract or other.
- Treat empirically with antibiotics while awaiting test results. Seek the advice of a microbiologist at an early stage regarding appropriate antibiotic therapy.
- The most common organism responsible for life-threatening infection in pregnant women is the beta-haemolytic *Streptococcus pyogenes* (Lancefield Group A); the most appropriate antibiotic for this is a combination of Tazocin (piperacillin and the beta-lactamase inhibitor tazobactam) and netilmicin.
- Beware of venous thromboembolism presenting as pyrexia.
- Watch for fetal tachycardia.

Action plan

☐ Send specimen for culture
   - vaginal swab
   - endocervical swab
   - midstream urine
   - blood
   - sputum and/or throat swab, if respiratory symptoms present.

☐ IV antibiotics: co-amoxiclav or cefuroxime will suffice as first-line therapy in women who are pyrexial but otherwise well. In severe cases, consider Tazocin (discuss with microbiologist).

☐ Inform paediatrician.

☐ Post-delivery, send the following for culture:
   - swabs from baby
   - placental swab.

Hepatitis B/C

Aim to reduce the chances of transmitting infection to the baby and/or staff. The risk of neonatal infection is variable (Table 5):

Table 5 *Risk of neonatal infection*

Infection type	Risk of neonatal infection (%)
Acute hepatitis B occurring between 28 weeks and term	80–90
Acute hepatitis earlier in pregnancy	10–30
HepBeAg positive	90
HepBeAg negative	30
Asymptomatic carrier	10

Action plan

☐ Admit into designated room.
☐ Check case notes for any instructions from the virologist regarding management.
☐ Universal precautions apply – wear disposable apron, gown, gloves, mask and spectacles.
☐ Attach 'Biohazard' label to blood specimens.
☐ For caesarean section and repair of episiotomy/perineal tear, consider use of blunt needles.
☐ Obtain cord blood for hepatitis B surface antigen (HBsAg) and e core antibody, HBeAb.
☐ Disinfect boots, bed and other material with antiseptic.
☐ Immunize baby.

- Do not use a fetal scalp electrode.
- Do not perform fetal blood sampling.

Hepatitis B/C is not a contraindication to breastfeeding.

Intrapartum antibiotic prophylaxis for group B streptococci

Principles

From 1% to 2% of babies born to women who carry group B streptococci (GBS) will develop clinical infection. Although this transmission rate is low, the fatality rate in affected babies is high (15–50%). Premature infants have a 10–15 times greater risk of acquiring GBS than do full-term infants.

Intrapartum antibiotic prophylaxis prevents vertical transmission and early-onset neonatal GBS.

Risk factors:

- labour at <35 weeks' gestation
- prolonged rupture of membranes (>18 hours)
- intrapartum pyrexia (>38°C, 100.4°F)
- previous delivery of infant with GBS
- GBS urinary tract infection
- previous high vaginal swab (HVS) showing GBS
- previous baby with neonatal GBS infection.

Action plan

For all women falling in the at-risk groups listed above:

☐ Send low vaginal swab for culture.
☐ Check for allergy to penicillin.
☐ Give penicillin 3 g IV load as soon as possible after onset of labour, then give 1.5 g every four hours until delivery. *If woman is allergic to penicillin, give clindamycin 900 mg IV every eight hours until delivered.*
☐ If GBS confirmed, flag the notes (a GBS sticker is available for this purpose) so that intrapartum antibiotic prophylaxis is not missed in the next pregnancy.
☐ If GBS is confirmed, ensure that the woman is informed fully. Emphasize the need for prophylactic antibiotics.

Intrapartum antibiotic prophylaxis is not required for women undergoing CS in the absence of labour and with intact membranes.

The baby should be managed as outlined in Figure 8 on p. 181.

Useful contact for patients: Group B Strep Support, PO Box 203, Haywards Heath, West Sussex RH16 1GF; Tel: 01444 416176; Web: www.gbss.org.uk

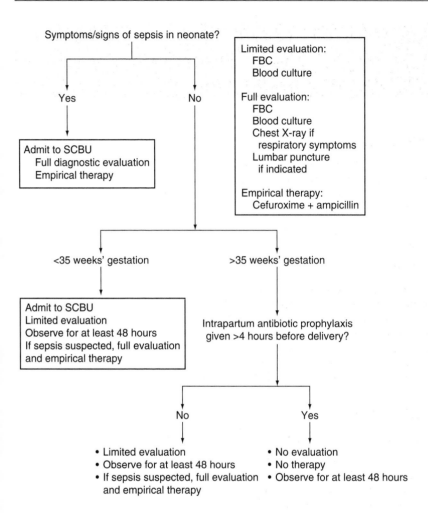

Figure 8 *Management of neonate whose mother received intrapartum antibiotic prophylaxis*

Genital herpes

About 90% of cases of genital herpes are caused by herpes simplex virus (HSV) type 2. It may present as painful vesicles or shallow ulcers, but there may be asymptomatic cervical lesions.

It may be a new (primary) infection or a recurrence. The risk of transmission to the baby is higher with primary infection (about 40%) than with recurrent infection (about 3%).

If a primary infection is present at term or in labour, then elective caesarean section should be offered; this reduces the risk of transmitting the infection to the baby.

Admission of a woman with vesicular lesion or history of genital herpes

- [ ] Examine vulva and cervix.
- [ ] Obtain cervical swab (and vulval swab if lesions present) for viral culture if diagnosis in doubt.
- [ ] If active herpes is present and fetal membranes are intact (or have just ruptured), offer caesarean section:
  - for primary (first-episode) infection, this is the recommended mode of delivery
  - for recurrent infection, the risk to the baby is small and must be weighed against the risk to the mother of a caesarean section.
- [ ] If more than four hours have elapsed since membranes ruptured, ascending infection is likely to have occurred and caesarean section is unlikely to reduce the risk of neonatal infection.
- [ ] Alert paediatricians.

> **!** It may be difficult to distinguish clinically between primary and recurrent genital herpes. If in doubt, treat as primary.

The following decision pathway is recommended (Figure 9).

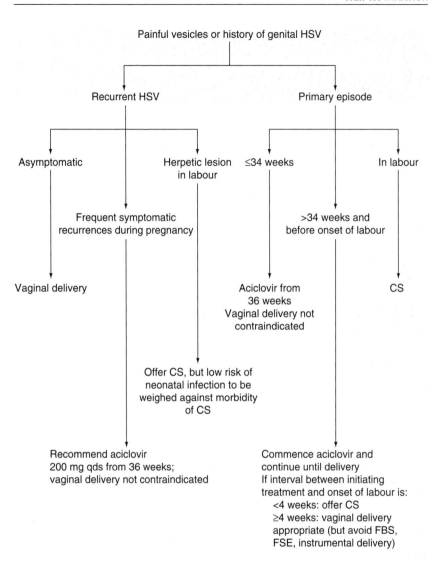

Figure 9 *Decision pathway for mode of delivery*

Human immunodeficiency virus

The following events increase the risk of vertical transmission of human immunodeficiency virus (HIV):

- vaginal delivery
- rupture of membranes >4 hours before delivery
- preterm delivery (particularly <34 weeks)
- use of fetal scalp electrode
- fetal scalp blood sampling
- chorioamnionitis
- breastfeeding
- high maternal viral load.

In women who have been treated appropriately with antiretroviral drugs, less than 10% of babies become infected with HIV.

Elective CS (usually at 38 weeks) with intact membranes reduces the risk of vertical transmission by at least 50%. However, if the mother has been on antiretroviral therapy and viral load is undetectable, then vaginal delivery will carry about the same risk of vertical transmission as elective CS.

Regional analgesia is not contraindicated.

Management of vaginal delivery

☐ Alert paediatrician.
☐ Treat any intercurrent infection.
☐ If on antiretroviral therapy, continue until delivery.
☐ Start zidovudine when in established labour or rupture of membranes is confirmed: initial dose 2 mg/kg IV over one hour (use weight at booking), followed by 1 mg/kg/hour until cord is clamped. To prepare the required dilution:
  - remove 100 ml from a 500-ml bag of 5% glucose, leaving 400 ml
  - take five vials each containing 20 ml of zidovudine at 10 mg/ml, and add this to the 400 ml of glucose 5%. This gives a solution of 1000 mg zidovudine in 500 ml, ie a concentration of 2 mg/ml. This may be kept for 24 hours if necessary
  - with this concentration, the *loading infusion rate* will be x ml/hour, where x is the weight (kg), and the *maintenance infusion rate* will be $0.5x$ ml/hour, where x is the weight (kg).
☐ If the woman is not on (or has only recently started) zidovudine, recommend

nevirapine 200 mg orally immediately at onset of labour, and start IV
zidovudine (see regime above).

☐ Cleanse vagina with chlorhexidine. Use Hibitane cream instead of KY Jelly.
☐ Avoid artificial rupture of membranes, if possible.
☐ Expedite delivery if there is inadequate uterine activity after spontaneous
rupture of membranes.
☐ Active phase of second stage of labour should not exceed one hour.

Other measures to reduce risk of vertical transmission

- The use of fetal scalp electrodes and fetal blood sampling are absolutely
contraindicated.
- Avoid episiotomy, if possible.
- If instrumental delivery is required, use forceps rather than ventouse.
- Clamp cord as quickly as possible after delivery.
- Suction of baby's mouth (*not trachea*) and nose immediately after delivery.
- Wash neonate immediately after birth in a warm bath.
- Recommend formula feeding. However, if the mother opts to breastfeed, then
respect her decision and support her.
- Administer antiretroviral medication to baby as prescribed (liaise with
paediatricians).

After delivery

- Arrange follow-up appointment in clinic.
- Maintain confidentiality.

Preparation for caesarean section

- Start zidovudine infusion four hours before operation. Initial dose 2 mg/kg IV
over one hour, followed by 1 mg/kg per hour until cord is clamped.
- Universal infection control measures apply.
- Use blunt needles.
- Use staples for skin.

Prelabour rupture of membranes

Preterm: assessment will have to be made as to the risk of HIV transmission
compared with the risk of premature delivery. This assessment should involve
obstetric, paediatric and infectious diseases staff. There is no known
contraindication to the use of short-term steroids to promote fetal lung maturity
in women with HIV.

At term: manage actively, aiming to keep the interval between rupture of
membranes and delivery less than four hours.

Cord blood

Cord blood should be taken for ultrasensitive HIV polymerase chain reaction (PCR), preferably in two EDTA bottles (one EDTA bottle will suffice if a sufficient sample to fill two bottles cannot be obtained). A clinical virology form must be completed, and 'ultrasensitive HIV PCR' must be written on the form.

To minimize needle-stick injuries, a segment of cord should be steadied using two pairs of forceps.

Care of the baby

- Skin-to-skin as soon as possible, unless declined by mother.
- Bathe baby.
- Administer vitamin K promptly, unless consent has been withheld.
- Antiretroviral therapy:
  - nevirapine 2 mg/kg orally, one dose only, within 72 hours of birth (the sooner the better), and zidovudine 2 mg/kg every six hours orally, starting within six hours of birth and continued for six weeks.
- If baby is premature or unable to tolerate oral medication, liaise with HIV physician for IV medication.

Infection control

- Any needlestick injury should be managed as stipulated in Trust policy.
- Standard personal protection equipment should be worn when undertaking any invasive procedures.

 Attach 'Biohazard' label to blood specimens.

Part V: Other obstetric emergencies

Cervical tear and paravaginal haematoma

Paravaginal haematoma may manifest as shock, in the absence of significant bleeding

- Examine in theatre under general anaesthesia or epidural analgesia.
- At examination under anaesthesia, ensure adequate exposure, with good lighting and an assistant.
- Assess whether blood transfusion is required (there is a tendency to underestimate blood loss).

Cervical tear

- Examine the cervix clockwise by serial clamping with sponge-holding forceps.
- Apex of tear must be identified. If apex cannot be seen, then a laparotomy is indicated.

Paravaginal haematoma

- Ensure complete evacuation of the haematoma. A large incision may be required.
- After evacuation and repair, a tight pack should be inserted in the vagina.
- Give IV antibiotic: co-amoxiclav or cefuroxime/metronidazole.

Rupture of the uterus

Early diagnosis depends on high index of suspicion.

Suspect ruptured uterus if there is:

- sudden sharp abdominal pain followed by cessation of uterine contractions
- abdominal tenderness
- fetal distress (usually bradycardia)
- vaginal bleeding
- maternal collapse
- haematuria.

 Any of the above in the presence of uterine scar is strongly suggestive of uterine rupture.

Action plan

- [ ] Call senior obstetrician and anaesthetist.
- [ ] Maintain airway with oxygen via facemask.
- [ ] Assess pulse and blood pressure.
- [ ] IV access (14G or larger).
- [ ] Full blood count and clotting screen, and cross-match six units.
- [ ] IV Hartmann's solution and blood transfusion as necessary.
- [ ] Cardiopulmonary resuscitation (CPR) if necessary.
- [ ] Continuous CTG (apply scalp electrode).
- [ ] Obtain consent for laparotomy, and possible hysterectomy, under general anaesthetic. The extent of the operation will depend on the extent of rupture, the amount of bleeding, and the patient's future reproductive intentions.
- [ ] IV co-amoxiclav or cefuroxime/metronidazole.

Preventive care

In contemporary practice, most women who suffer a ruptured uterus have had a previous CS or an oxytocic drug, or both. All women undergoing a trial of vaginal delivery after CS should be informed of the risk of scar rupture (about 1–2%).

In the presence of a uterine scar, prostaglandin or Syntocinon infusion should be used only with the prior approval of a consultant obstetrician, and the woman must be informed of the threefold increase in risk of scar rupture.

Induction of labour in women with a previous CS should be in accordance with the protocol on p. 86.

Vaginal birth after CS should be managed as outlined on pp. 80–81.

With Syntocinon induction or augmentation of labour, there should be continuous electronic fetal monitoring, and as much attention should be paid to the tocograph as to the cardiograph.

Shoulder dystocia

Risk factors include:

- large baby
- diabetes
- previous shoulder dystocia
- secondary arrest after 8 cm cervical dilatation.

 50% of shoulder dystocia occurs in normal-sized babies.
More than 90% of macrosomic babies do not have dystocia.

Risks to mother and baby include:

- birth asphyxia
- fractures
- brachial plexus damage
- perineal trauma.

When shoulder dystocia is anticipated:

- discuss with the woman
- give epidural early in labour
- deliver in lithotomy position
- registrar to be present at delivery
- adequate episiotomy.

Action plan

☐ **H** Call for *help*: senior obstetrician, second midwife, paediatrician and anaesthetist. A glance at the clock as you call for help or start manoeuvres is helpful. Nominate someone to record timing and sequence of events.

☐ **E** *Evaluate* for *episiotomy*.

☐ **L** *Legs*: place in *lithotomy* position, with full flexion and abduction of the hips – the thighs should touch the abdomen. (This is McRobert's manoeuvre; it requires two assistants.) Attempt delivery in this position for 60 seconds. If this fails, the woman remains in this position while the next manoeuvre is performed.

☐ **P** *Pressure*: apply suprapubic pressure (to the anterior shoulder), directed sideways, towards the anterior surface of the fetal chest. Initially pressure is applied continuously; if this is unsuccessful, try a rocking motion.

Downward traction is applied on baby's head and neck, without lateral flexion of the neck.

If the above measures fail to deliver the shoulder (about one in 10 cases):

☐ **E** *Enter* manoeuvres:
  – insert fingers behind anterior shoulder and push it toward the baby's chest
  – Woods' screw manoeuvre – apply pressure with two fingers in front of the posterior shoulder and two fingers behind the anterior shoulder
  – reverse Woods' screw – apply pressure with fingers behind the posterior shoulder.

☐ **R** *Remove* the posterior arm. Deliver the posterior arm by following the humerus up to the elbow and flexing it. Grasp the wrist and sweep the arm across the chest until it is delivered.

☐ **R** *Roll* the woman on to her hands and knees. Deliver the posterior arm by downward traction.

If the above drill is not successful and the baby is still alive, try either replacement of the baby's head and CS, with the aid of tocolytic and constant pressure on the head, or perform symphysiotomy.

If the baby is dead, cleidotomy may be performed.

☐ Carefully examine the genital tract for damage after delivery.
☐ Document manoeuvres performed and time taken.
☐ Review events with the woman and her partner.

Cord prolapse

Cord prolapse is when the umbilical cord slips below the presenting part, with ruptured membranes.

It should always be excluded when spontaneous rupture of the membranes occurs and when amniotomy is performed.

Diagnosis may be suggested by sudden abnormalities on the CTG.

Risk factors:

- breech presentation
- high head at onset of labour
- multiple pregnancy
- polyhydramnios
- preterm labour.

Action plan

☐ Ring emergency bell.
☐ Summon registrar, anaesthetist and paediatrician (fast bleep ....).
☐ Summon anaesthetic practitioner
  – tel .....
  – after hours .....
  – bleep .....
☐ Keep fingers in the vagina to push the presenting part above and away from the cord. If necessary, feel for pulsation but avoid unnecessary handling.
☐ Tilt the head of the bed down or place the patient in the knee/chest (all-fours) position. If epidural is sited, place woman in left lateral position.
☐ Move woman to theatre immediately.
☐ If cord pulsation not palpable, use CTG and/or scan to ascertain status of fetus.
☐ Explain to woman and her partner what is happening.
☐ Deliver by caesarean section unless:
  – cervix is fully dilated and presenting part is below the ischial spines (in which case ventouse or forceps delivery), or
  – baby is not alive.
☐ Umbilical cord pH.
☐ Discuss event with the woman and her partner.
☐ Documentation: chronological account of events and management.

If for any reason delivery is delayed, fill the bladder with 500 ml normal saline. This relieves cord compression directly as well as indirectly (by inhibiting uterine contractions) – but don't forget to empty the bladder before proceeding with CS.

Anaphylaxis

Presentation: itching, flushing, rash, nausea, vomiting, breathlessness, wheezing, oedema, tachycardia, hypotension, respiratory or cardiac collapse.

Action plan

- [ ] Summon help.
- [ ] Discontinue/remove offending agent.
- [ ] Assess airways, breathing and circulation, and commence basic life support if appropriate.
- [ ] Raise the feet to help restore blood pressure.
- [ ] Oxygen by bag and mask.
- [ ] Administer 0.5 mg adrenaline (epinephrine) IM (ie 0.5 ml of 1:1000 injection). Repeat every 10 minutes until blood pressure and pulse are normal or help arrives.
- [ ] Monitor vital signs and O_2 saturation.
- [ ] 14FG IV cannula.
- [ ] IV infusion – Gelofusine/Haemaccel.
- [ ] Check arterial blood gases.
- [ ] Chlorpheniramine 10 mg IV, slow infusion.
- [ ] Hydrocortisone 100 mg IV immediately.
- [ ] Aminophylline 250 mg IV over 20 minutes.
- [ ] Continuous electronic fetal monitoring, if prenatal.

Inverted uterus

Uterine inversion is when the fundus prolapses into the body of the uterus and beyond. This may occur spontaneously or as a result of mismanagement of the third stage of labour. It causes severe pain and may result in shock without evidence of bleeding. Haemorrhagic shock could occur if inversion has followed uterine atony.

Rapid colloid infusion may fail to improve the woman's condition, and care should be taken to avoid fluid overload.

Action plan

- ☐ If woman is in shock, assess airway, breathing and circulation; summon help and commence basic life support if appropriate.
- ☐ Exclude submucous fibroid (uterus will be palpable abdominally).
- ☐ Maintain IV access (18G cannula), and give Hartmann's solution.
- ☐ Full blood count.
- ☐ Cross-match four units of blood.
- ☐ Reduce the inverted uterus.
- ☐ Commence Syntocinon infusion, 40 units in 500 ml 5% dextrose following successful reduction.

Reduction of the inversion
Manual reduction

If the inversion occurs during delivery, it may be possible to replace the uterus immediately with Entonox or IM pethidine. If an effective epidural analgesia is already in place, then this could be adequate. In all other circumstances, and *particularly if the woman is in shock*, reduction of an inverted uterus should be performed under a general anaesthetic.

If the placenta has not separated, replace the uterus and commence Syntocinon infusion (40 units in 500 ml Hartmann's solution), then perform manual removal of the placenta. Do not attempt to remove the placenta before replacing the uterus.

Hydrostatic reduction

- ■ Exclude vaginal tear and rupture of the uterus before using this technique.

- Use *warm* saline (start with 1 l bag) via a wide-bore giving set. The bag should be about 1 m above the patient (this gives a hydrostatic pressure of 100 cm H_2O). Do not use hypotonic fluid.
- The accoucheur covers the vaginal introitus with his/her hands, or with a 6-cm silastic ventouse cup is applied to the end of a wide-bore giving set to provide a seal.
- *A general anaesthetic is not mandatory.*
- If the placenta has not separated, then replace the uterus and commence Syntocinon infusion (40 units in 500 ml Hartmann's), then perform manual removal of the placenta.
- Keep a record of the amounts of fluid infused into the vagina and released from it.

 Do not attempt to remove the placenta before replacing the uterus, as doing so could increase haemorrhage, shock and intravasation of fluid.

Sometimes it will be necessary to administer a tocolytic. Rarely, it may be necessary to perform laparotomy and reduction from above.

Acute inversion may be complicated by pulmonary oedema from excessive IV fluids or, in cases of hydrostatic replacement, from fluid intravasation.

Discuss management of third stage of labour in next pregnancy.

Amniotic fluid embolism

This condition may occur suddenly in labour, at caesarean section, or soon after delivery. The mortality rate is about 60–80%. Morbidity in survivors is high. Cardiovascular collapse and respiratory symptoms are the most common initial presentations.

A high index of suspicion could be life-saving. This rare condition must be suspected if there is:

- disorientation/agitation/delirium
- sudden shock (cardiovascular collapse)
- respiratory distress
- cyanosis
- fetal distress
- coma
- coagulopathy.

If the above occur during labour or caesarean section or within 30 minutes postpartum and there is no other explanation (ie the differential diagnoses have been excluded), then a clinical diagnosis of amniotic fluid embolism can be made.

Differential diagnoses include:

- pulmonary embolism
- myocardial infarction
- Mendelson syndrome
- cerebrovascular accident
- total spinal
- septic shock
- substance abuse
- placental abruption.
- eclampsia.

Management

- [ ] Summon help.
- [ ] Commence basic life support.
- [ ] Full blood count.
- [ ] Coagulation profile: PT, APPT, fibrinogen.
- [ ] FDP/D-dimer.
- [ ] Urea and electrolytes.

- [ ] Liver function tests.
- [ ] IV access; intravenous fluids.
- [ ] Cross-match four units of blood.
- [ ] Chest X-ray.
- [ ] Ventilation–perfusion scan.
- [ ] ECG.
- [ ] Pulse oximetry.
- [ ] Automated blood pressure monitoring.
- [ ] CVP; arterial catheter.
- [ ] Urinary catheter.
- [ ] CTG, if undelivered.
- [ ] Contact consultant haematologist immediately – do not wait until coagulopathy is evident. Transfusion of fresh frozen plasma, cryoprecipitate and platelets as advised by haematologist. Liaise with consultant anaesthetist.
- [ ] Transfer to ITU as soon as possible. If undelivered, an urgent caesarean section should be performed before transfer.

Delivery should occur within 5 minutes of cardiac arrest, if there is no response to initial resuscitation (neonatal outcome dependent on short cardiac arrest-to-delivery interval).

Other aspects of management are as outlined for sudden collapse, pp. 200–201.

Amniotic fluid embolism register

Entry criteria:

- acute hypotension or cardiac arrest
- acute hypoxia (dyspnoea, cyanosis or respiratory arrest)
- coagulopathy
- onset of all the above during labour or caesarean section, or within 30 minutes of delivery
- no other clinical condition or potential explanation for symptoms and signs.

All cases meeting the above criteria, whether the patient survives or not, should be reported to Derek Tufnell, Bradford Royal Infirmary, Duckworth Lane, Bradford BD9 6RJ; Tel: 01274 364520.

Sudden maternal collapse

Possible causes include:

- postpartum haemorrhage (possibly concealed in broad ligament or paravaginal haematoma)
- sepsis
- pneumothorax
- pulmonary embolus
- amniotic fluid embolism
- cardiac arrhythmia
- inverted uterus
- myocardial infarction
- left ventricular failure
- hypoglycaemia
- diabetic ketoacidosis
- cerebrovascular accident
- drug reaction
- anaphylaxis
- thyroid crisis
- uterine rupture
- peripartum cardiomyopathy
- ruptured aneurysm.

Management

☐ Assess airway, breathing and circulation.

☐ Crash call (see p. 3) and commence basic life support if appropriate; otherwise, turn to left lateral position.

☐ If cardiopulmonary resuscitation (CPR) is required, ensure that pressure on the inferior vena cava by the pregnant uterus is relieved by means of a wedge under the side of the woman.

☐ Examine for signs of vaginal bleeding, peritonitis and breathing difficulties.

☐ Consider intubation (by anaesthetist, with cricoid pressure by assistant), to reduce risk of pulmonary aspiration.

☐ Give oxygen using bag and mask, 6 l/min

☐ IV infusion Haemaccel or Gelofusine.

☐ If in pain give IM pethidine 50–100 mg immediately.

Investigations

☐ Full blood count.
☐ Urea and electrolytes.
☐ Liver function tests.
☐ Coagulation screen.
☐ Blood gases.
☐ Group and cross-match.
☐ ECG.
☐ Portable chest X-ray.

If patient is diabetic, check blood sugar with glucometer and then give infusion of 50 ml 50% dextrose and insert urinary catheter. Inform on-call medical registrar.

If resuscitation has been unsuccessful after 5 minutes, proceed to CS – not only to save the baby but also to increase the mother's chances of survival.

Latex allergy

For treatment of anaphylaxis, see p. 195.

Risk factors:

- history of multiple surgical procedures
- history of atopy (hay fever, asthma, dermatitis, food allergy)
- previous anaphylactic episode of unknown cause, particularly if associated with surgery or dental treatment
- occupational exposure to latex.

A latex-free pack for emergency use should always be available on the delivery suite.

Care of the woman allergic to latex

- Labour should be conducted in a latex-free room.
- Case notes, patient identification band and room door should carry warning of latex allergy.
- Prepare a trolley with latex-free gloves, catheters, surgical tape, IV equipment and tourniquets for possible emergency use.
- Inform anaesthetist.
- Management of IV drugs:
  - draw up in latex-free syringes
  - do not reconstitute or inject through rubber bungs.
- Beware of latex blood pressure cuffs.
- Prepare back-up theatre (to be latex-free) in case an emergency CS is required. Minimum dust-settling time is two hours.
- Drugs used to treat allergic reactions ready for use.

The following should not be used or left exposed in the care of a woman who is allergic to latex:

- latex gloves
- Foley catheter
- Entonox rubber tubing
- elasticated straps for CTG monitor
- rubber tourniquet
- sphygmomanometer tubing
- Elastoplast
- rubber mattress covers on theatre tables
- other rubber products.

Theatre (elective or emergency procedure)

Only essential personnel to be in theatre.

Put up notices on theatre doors, marking the theatre as a latex-free room, and keep the doors shut.

Part VI: Stillbirths and congenital abnormalities

Checklist for fetal loss at 13–23 weeks

Parents

- ☐ Parents given the opportunity to see and hold the fetus.
- ☐ Has a minister of religion been requested?
- ☐ Parents offered a photograph.
- ☐ Parents informed about the choice of hospital or private funeral. Information leaflet provided.
- ☐ Post-mortem examination discussed:
  - – has consent been given?
  - – has consent *not* been given?
- ☐ Appropriate bereavement pack provided.
- ☐ Anti-D given/not required.
- ☐ Follow-up appointment made.
- ☐ Woman seen by doctor before discharge home.

Communication

- ☐ Arrange suppression of mail for parent education classes, antenatal clinic and other antenatal activities.
- ☐ Antenatal clinic informed of fetal loss.
- ☐ GP informed by telephone and letter.

Forms/administration

- ☐ Complete all forms per local protocol.
- ☐ Fetal loss register completed.
- ☐ Arrangements made for transport to mortuary.

Intrauterine fetal demise

Principles

- Be sure of the diagnosis before informing the patient.
- Keep the woman and her partner fully informed of what is happening.
- Show a caring attitude but also give the woman and her partner the time and space they require.
- The investigations performed will depend on whether there was an obvious cause of fetal loss.
- The issue of consent for post-mortem examination is probably best brought up when discussing the cause of death.

Diagnosis (if not made before admission)

First indication might be absence of fetal movement or inability to pick up fetal heart tones.

Obstetrician should perform ultrasound scan. If fetal heart pulsation is not seen, ask for a formal/reported scan by ultrasonographer. Inform the woman that fetal heart pulsation has not been seen but that a further scan is required and will be performed as soon as possible. Inform consultant.

The senior obstetrician should discuss diagnosis and management with patient. Decisions must be made regarding when and how to deliver the baby. Administer mifepristone 200 mg orally, under supervision.

The GP, community midwife and health visitor should be informed, and antenatal appointments cancelled.

Action plan

Ideally, mifepristone should have been administered 36–48 hours before admission.

☐ Admit into designated room.
☐ Discuss tests, including post-mortem examination of the baby.
☐ Provide information booklets on funeral arrangements and post-mortem examination, including *Examination of the Body after Death – Information About Post-mortem Examination for Relatives*. London: Royal College of Pathologists, March 2000 (accessible at http://www.rcpath.org/resources/pdf/patients_leaflet.pdf).

☐ Document consent for tests.
☐ Induction of labour – see below.
☐ Investigations – see below.
☐ Consider antibiotic treatment.
☐ Discuss funeral arrangements – private or hospital burial – or disposal by pathology laboratory.
☐ Offer counselling and provide details of support groups.
☐ If possible, avoid artificial rupture of membranes (risk of infection).
☐ Ask parents if they wish to name the baby. Record name in notes.
☐ Examine baby: wash, weigh, measure and label; check for abnormalities.
☐ Dress the baby (after examination always keep baby clothed).
☐ Parents allowed to see/hold baby for as long as they wish.
☐ Photograph taken of baby.
☐ Stillbirth certificate completed and signed.
☐ Prescribe medication to suppress lactation:
  – cabergoline 1 mg orally, single dose
  – bromocriptine 2.5 mg bd for 14 days is a less expensive option but carries more risks; it should not be given to women with hypertension, coronary artery disease or any mental disorder.
☐ Arrange follow-up appointment.

Investigations

Maternal blood tests:

☐ Full blood count (pink EDTA bottle, general blood card).
☐ HbA1c (glycated haemoglobin).
☐ Blood group antibodies (universal bottle, pink sheet).
☐ Kleihauer test (pink EDTA bottle, general blood card).
☐ Lupus anticoagulant (two green coagulation and one universal bottle, scripted request on general blood card).
☐ Anticardiolipin antibodies.
☐ Coagulation screen.
☐ TORCH screen (universal bottle, virology card): *Toxoplasma*, rubella, cytomegalovirus and hepatitis antibodies.
☐ Parvovirus B19 screen (universal bottle, virology card).
☐ Chromosome analysis, if not known (lithium heparin, ie orange bottle, genetics card).
☐ Any other clinically indicated blood test.
☐ Urine for drugs screen, if there is a suspicion of drug misuse.
☐ Vaginal swab (taken during routine examination before inducing labour).
☐ Placenta:
  – swab for culture
  – send to pathology (histology) in bucket with formalin and histology card.

Fetus tests:

☐ Full-depth fetal skin biopsy (0.5 cm³), taken from the axilla, for cytogenetics/fluorescent *in situ* hybridization (FISH)
  – do not clean skin before biopsy
  – skin biopsy culture usually fails in macerated stillbirth.
☐ Send placenta for histology tests.
☐ Cord or cardiac blood sample (at least 0.5 ml into a 1–2-ml lithium heparin paediatric tube), for FBC, chromosome analysis, culture.
☐ Swabs from nose, throat, ear and umbilicus.
☐ Photographs.
☐ Post-mortem.
☐ X-ray of baby.

Induction of labour

Ensure that fetal lie is longitudinal before induction of labour. If lie is abnormal, then senior obstetrician to discuss version with the woman.

If fetal demise has occurred in mid-trimester, follow algorithm on pp. 212–213.

If in the third trimester, assess cervix and proceed as follows:

- *Cervix favourable:* perform amniotomy and commence Syntocinon infusion.
- *Cervix unfavourable for amniotomy but cervical score >5:* insert prostaglandin E_2 (PGE_2) gel 1 mg. Repeat four hours later if cervix remains unfavourable for amniotomy.
- *Cervical score <5, and no contraindications to gemeprost:* insert a gemeprost 1-mg pessary; repeat every three hours until labour is induced or amniotomy is feasible.
- *Cervical score <5 and gemeprost contraindicated:* use prostaglandin E_2 gel 2 mg. If required, a further dose of prostaglandin E_2 gel 1 mg may be given four hours later.

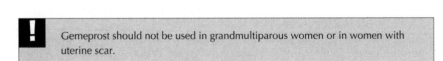

! Gemeprost should not be used in grandmultiparous women or in women with uterine scar.

If cervix remains unfavourable for amniotomy despite two doses of PGE_2 gel, consider using extra-amniotic prostaglandin (see below).

If labour is not induced after five doses of gemeprost, allow 12–24 hours then commence extra-amniotic prostaglandin as follows:

☐ One ampoule containing 5 mg of PGE_2 dissolved in 0.5 ml ethanol and 50 ml of saline. This gives a 100 µg/ml solution.

☐ Obtain a 12–14FG Foley catheter with a 30 ml balloon. Fill the dead space with 3 ml of the solution you have prepared.

☐ Under aseptic conditions, insert the catheter through the cervix and inflate the balloon.

☐ Start infusion at an initial rate of 1 ml/hour, increasing to 2 ml/hour if there is no uterine response after four hours.

☐ When the catheter falls out, amniotomy may be performed.

 Note that PGE$_2$ potentiates the effect of Syntocinon on the uterus.

If labour is not induced despite the measures described above, further management will be determined by the consultant, based on the circumstances and preferences of the woman.

For twin delivery after 24 weeks when one twin is known to have died *in utero* before viability: the dead twin has to be registered as a stillbirth; it is assigned the gestational age of the live twin.

Support group:

Stillbirth and Neonatal Death Society (SANDS), 28 Portland Place, London W1B 1LY. Helpline: 020 7436 5881 (10:00–15:00 GMT, Monday to Friday); Office: 020 7436 7940 (10:00–17:00 GMT, Monday to Friday); Fax: 020 7436 3715; Web: www.uk-sands.org

Mid-trimester termination of pregnancy for fetal abnormality

The principles of management are as outlined for intrauterine fetal demise (pp. 208–211). Ensure that the statutory forms for termination of pregnancy have been completed.

Induction of labour

Follow protocol on p. 214.

Investigations

These will depend on the nature of the abnormality.

Prenatal diagnosis of chromosomal abnormality

☐ Full-depth fetal skin biopsy (0.5 cm³) for cytogenetics/fluorescent *in situ* hybridization (FISH).
☐ Sample of cord (2–3 cm in length) and sample of placental membrane from around the cord-insertion site.
☐ Cord or cardiac blood sample (at least 0.5 ml into a 1–2 ml lithium heparin paediatric tube).

Send solid specimen in dry pot – *do not use formalin*. If transport has to be delayed overnight, store at 4°C; *do not freeze*. Ensure container is labelled properly.

Ultrasound scan diagnosis of structural abnormality or external appearance suggestive of aneuploidy

☐ Full-depth fetal skin biopsy (0.5 cm³) for cytogenetics/FISH.
☐ Sample of cord (2–3 cm in length) and sample of placental membrane from around the cord-insertion site.
☐ Cord or cardiac blood sample (at least 0.5 ml into a 1–2 ml lithium heparin paediatric tube).

Send solid specimen in dry pot – *do not use formalin*. If transport has to be delayed overnight, store at 4°C; *do not freeze*. Ensure container is labelled properly.

Scan diagnosis of neural tube defect, with no other malformation or recurrences in family

Cytogenetic diagnosis is not routinely required in these cases.

Genetic examination of fetuses and samples

Only fetuses (and samples) aborted in the following circumstances should be sent to the laboratory:

- prenatal diagnosis of chromosome abnormality
- scan diagnosis of structural abnormality (in the case of neural tube defects, those with other abnormalities or where there has been recurrence in the family)
- miscarriage where the baby has obvious malformations.

Support group:

Antenatal Results and Choices (formerly Support After Termination for Anomaly, SAFTA), 73–75 Charlotte Place, London W1P 1LB. Tel: 0207 631 0280 (Administration), 0207 631 0285 (Helpline); Email: arcsafta@aol.com

Protocol for medical termination of mid-trimester pregnancy

As part of the process of obtaining consent for this procedure, an information leaflet should be provided. The leaflet should include contact details.

☐ Woman takes one tablet (200 mg) of mifepristone, witnessed by staff.

☐ Observe for one hour. If vomiting occurs, give prochlorperazine (Stemetil) 12.5 mg IM and repeat mifepristone.

☐ Discharge home; discharge information to include contact telephone number.

☐ 36–48 hours later, woman attends ward and procedure is explained again.

☐ Misoprostol 800 μg (or gemeprost 1 mg) inserted into the posterior fornix.

☐ If fetus/products have not been expelled, give oral misoprostol 400 μg every four hours (or gemeprost 1 mg pessary every three hours) up to a maximum of four doses.

☐ Analgesia given as required (co-codamol every four hours or diamorphine 5–10 mg IM every four hours).

☐ Record blood pressure, pulse and temperature hourly.

☐ If first course of treatment was successful and woman is in stable condition, discharge home, inform GP, and confirm follow-up arrangements.

☐ If first course of treatment was not successful, allow 12 hours from last dose before commencing second course of gemeprost pessaries, as above.

Contraindications

The use of mifepristone is contraindicated in the following:

- allergy to mifepristone
- chronic renal failure
- long-term corticosteroid therapy
- clotting disorders or anticoagulant therapy
- anaemia ([Hb] <8.5 g/dl)
- smoker aged ≥35 years
- suspected ectopic pregnancy.

The use of misoprostol or gemeprost is contraindicated in the following:

- allergy to prostaglandins
- severe asthma.

Caution

Use mifepristone with caution in the following:

- asthma
- chronic obstructive airway disease
- cardiovascular disease
- renal failure
- liver failure
- prosthetic heart valves.

Use misoprostol and gemeprost with caution in the following:

- cerebrovascular disease
- coronary artery disease
- severe peripheral vascular disease, including hypertension.

Further reading

Caesarean section

Lucas DN, Yentis SM, Kinsella SM, *et al.* Urgency of caesarean section: a new classification. *J R Soc Med* 2000; **93**: 346–50.

NHS Litigation Authority. Criterion 3.2.5. In: *Clinical Negligence Scheme for Trusts Clinical Risk Management Standards for Maternity Services*. London: NHS Litigation Authority, 2002.

Small F, Hofmeyr GJ. Antibiotic prophylaxis for cesarean section. Cochrane Review. In: *The Cochrane Library* Issue 3, 2002. Oxford: Update Software.

Thomas J, Paranjothy S. Royal College of Obstetricians and Gynaecologists Clinical Effectiveness Support Unit. *National Sentinel Caesarean Section Audit Report*. London: RCOG Press, 2001.

Wilkinson C, Enkin MW. Manual removal of placenta at caesarean section. Cochrane Review. In: *The Cochrane Library* Issue 3, 2002. Oxford: Update Software.

Recovery of obstetric patients

Fairfield MC, Bland D, Mushambi MC. Post-anaesthesia recovery care on the labour ward. *Int J Obstet Anesth* 1997; **6**: 153–5.

NHS Litigation Authority. Criterion 4.1.4. In: *Clinical Negligence Scheme for Trusts Clinical Risk Management Standards For Maternity Services*. London: NHS Litigation Authority, 2002.

UK Health Departments. *Report on Confidential Enquiries into Maternal Deaths in the United Kingdom 1988–1990*. London: HMSO, 1994.

The Association of Anaesthetists of Great Britain and Ireland. *Immediate postanaesthetic recovery*. London: The Association of Anaesthetists of Great Britain and Ireland, September 2002. www.aagbi.org

The Association of Anaesthetists of Great Britain and Ireland and The Obstetric Anaesthetists Association. *Guidelines for obstetric anaesthesia services*. London: The Association of Anaesthetists of Great Britain and Ireland and The Obstetric Anaesthetists Association, September 1998.

High-dependency care

Collis RE. Anaesthesia for caesarean section: general anaesthesia. In: Collis R, Plaat F, Urquhart J (eds). *Textbook of Obstetric Anaesthesia*. London: Greenwich Medical Media, 2002, Chapter 8, pp. 113–31.

Dhond GR, Ridley SA. Intensive and high dependency care of the obstetric patient. In: Collis R, Plaat F, Urquhart J (eds). *Textbook of Obstetric Anaesthesia*. London: Greenwich Medical Media, 2002, Chapter 15, pp. 235–50.

Instrumental delivery

Clements RV. Operative obstetrics. In: Clements RV (ed). *Risk Management and Litigation in Obstetrics and Gynaecology*. London: RSM Press, 2001, pp. 205–42.

Edozien LC, Williams J, Chattopadhyay I, Hirsch PJ. Failed instrumental delivery: How safe is the use of a second instrument? *J Obstet Gynaecol* 1999; **19**: 460–62.

Johanson R, Menon V. Soft versus rigid vacuum extractor cups for assisted vaginal delivery. Cochrane Review. In: *The Cochrane Library*, Issue 2, 2003. Oxford: Update Software.

Murphy DJ, Liebling RE, Patel R, *et al.* Cohort study of operative delivery in the second stage of labour and standard of obstetric care. *Br J Obstet Gynaecol* 2003; **110**: 610–15.

Royal College of Obstetricians and Gynaecologists. Instrumental Vaginal Delivery. Clinical Green Top Guideline no. 26. London: Royal College of Obstetricians and Gynaecologists, 2000.

Sadan O, Ginath S, Gomel A, et al. Vacuum application through a nonfully dilated cervix: a viable option. *Arch Gynecol Obstet* 2003; **268**: 281–3.

Trial of vaginal delivery after caesarean section

American College of Obstetricians and Gynecologists. Vaginal birth after previous cesarean delivery. Practice Bulletin No. 5. Washington, DC: American College of Obstetricians and Gynecologists, 1999.

Chazotte C, Madden R, Cohen WR. Labor patterns in women with previous cesareans. *Obstet Gynecol* 1990; **75**: 350–55.

Khan KS, Rizvi A. The partograph in the management of labor following caesarean section. *Int J Gynecol Obstet* 1995; **50**: 151–7.

Induction of labour

National Institute for Clinical Excellence. Guidelines for Induction of Labour. In: *Summary of Guidance Issued to the NHS in England and Wales*, issue 6. London; NICE April 2003 pp. 84–93.

Royal College of Obstetricians and Gynaecologists. Induction of Labour. Evidence-based Clinical Guideline no. 9. London: Royal College of Obstetricians and Gynaecologists, 2001.

Preterm prelabour rupture of fetal membranes

Kenyon S, Boulvain M, Neilson J. Antibiotics for preterm premature rupture of membranes. Cochrane Review. In: *The Cochrane Library*, Issue 2, 2003. Oxford: Update Software.

Kenyon S, Taylor D, Tarnow-Mordi W. Broad spectrum antibiotics for preterm, prelabour rupture of fetal membranes: the ORACLE I randomised trial. *Lancet* 2001; **357**: 979–88.

Lamont RF. Recent evidence associated with the condition of preterm prelabour rupture of the membranes. *Curr Opin Obstet Gynecol* 2003; **15**: 91–9.

Preterm uterine contractions

King J, Flenady V. Prophylactic antibiotics for inhibiting preterm labour with intact membranes. Cochrane Review. In: *The Cochrane Library*, Issue 2, 2003. Oxford: Update Software.

Morales WJ, Smith SG, Angel JA, et al. Efficacy and safety of indomethacin versus ritodrine in the management of preterm labour: a randomized study. *Obstet Gynecol* 1989; **74**: 567–72.

Moutquin JM, Sherman D, Cohen HM, et al. Double-blind, randomised, controlled trial of atosiban and ritodrine in the treatment of preterm labour: a multicenter effectiveness and safety study. *Am J Obstet Gynecol* 2000; **182**: 1191–9.

Papatsonis DN, van Geijn HP, Ader HJ, et al. Nifedipine and ritodrine in the management of preterm labour: a randomised multicentre trial. *Obstet Gynecol* 1997; **90**: 230–34.

Royal College of Obstetricians and Gynaecologists. Tocolytic Drugs for Women in Preterm Labour. Clinical Green Top Guideline no. 1b. London: Royal College of Obstetricians and Gynaecologists, 2002.

Worldwide Atosiban versus Beta-agonists Study Group. Effectiveness and safety of the oxytocin antagonist atosiban versus beta-adrenergic agonists in the treatment of preterm labour. *Br J Obstet Gynaecol* 2001; **108**: 133–42.

Antenatal corticosteroid therapy

Crowley P. Prophylactic corticosteroids for preterm birth. Cochrane Review. In: *The Cochrane Library*, Issue 3, 2002. Oxford: Update Software.

Royal College of Obstetricians and Gynaecologists. Antenatal Corticosteroids to Prevent Respiratory Distress Syndrome. Clinical Green Top Guideline no. 7. London: Royal College of Obstetricians and Gynaecologists, 1999.

Deliveries at the lower margin of viability

American Academy of Pediatrics Committee on Fetus and Newborn. American College of Obstetricians and Gynecologists Committee on Obstetric Practice. Perinatal care at the threshold of viability. *Pediatrics* 1995; **96**: 974–6.

British Association of Perinatal Medicine. Fetuses and Newborn Infants at the Threshold of Viability: A Framework for Practice. Memorandum. London: British Association of Perinatal Medicine, 1999.

Costeloe K, Hennessy E, Gibson AT *et al*. The EPICure study: outcomes to discharge from hospital for infants born at the threshold of viability. *Paediatrics* 2000; **106**: 659–71.

Rennie JM. Perinatal management at the lower margin of viability. *Arch Dis Child Fetal Neonatal Ed* 1996; **74**: F214–18.

Royal College of Obstetricians and Gynaecologists. *A Consideration of the Law and Ethics in Relation to Late Termination for Fetal Abnormality*. London: Royal College of Obstetricians and Gynaecologists, 1998.

Multiple pregnancy

Baskett TF. *Essential Management of Obstetric Emergencies*, 3rd edn. Bristol: Clinical Press, 1999, Chapter 15, pp. 151–8.

Belfort MA. Intravenous nitroglycerin as a tocolytic agent for intrapartum external cephalic version. *S Afr Med J* 1993; **83**: 656–7.

Dufour PH, Vinatier S, Vanderstichele S *et al*. Intravenous nitroglycerin for intrapartum podalic version of the second twin in transverse lie. *Obstet Gynecol* 1998; **92**: 416–9.

Hofmeyr GJ, Drakeley AJ. Delivery of twins. In: Neilson JP (ed). *Multiple Pregnancy. Baillière's Clinical Obstetrics and Gynaecology,* Volume 12. London: Baillière Tindall, 1998 pp. 91–108.

Malpresentation

Singh S, Paterson-Brown S. Malpresentations in labour. *Curr Obstet Gynaecol* 2003; **13**: 300–6.

Occipitoposterior position

Hofmeyr GJ, Kulier R. Hands/knees posture in late pregnancy or labour for fetal malposition (lateral or posterior). Cochrane Review. In: *The Cochrane Library*, Issue 2, 2003. Oxford: Update Software.

Breech presentation

Grant A. Elective vs selective caesarean delivery of the small baby. Cochrane Review. In: *The Cochrane Library*, Issue 2, 2003. Oxford: Update Software.

Hannah ME, Hannah WJ, Hewson SA, *et al.*, for the Term Breech Trial Collaborative Group. Planned caesarean section versus planned vaginal birth for breech presentation at term: a randomised multicentre trial. *Lancet* 2000; **356**: 1375–83.

Nwosu EC, Walkinshaw S, Chia P, *et al*. Undiagnosed breech. *Br J Obstet Gynaecol* 1993; **100**: 531–5.

Royal College of Obstetricians and Gynaecologists. The Management of Breech Presentation. Clinical Green Top Guideline no. 20. London: Royal College of Obstetricians and Gynaecologists, 2001.

External cephalic version

Ben-Haroush A, Perri T, Bar J *et al*. Mode of delivery following successful external cephalic version. *Am J Perinatol* 2002; **19**: 355–60.

Bujold E, Marquette GP, Ferreira E *et al*. Sublingual nitroglycerin versus intravenous ritodrine as tocolytic for external cephalic version: a double-blinded randomized trial. *Am J Obstet Gynecol* 2003; **188**: 1454–7.

De Meeus JB, Ellia F, Magnin G. External cephalic version after previous caesarean section: a series of 38 cases. *Eur J Obstet Gynecol Reprod Biol* 1998; **81**: 65–8.

Ferguson JE 2nd, Dyson DC. Intrapartum external cephalic version. *Am J Obstet Gynecol* 1985; **152**: 297–8.

Hofmeyr GJ. Interventions to help external cephalic version for breech presentation at term. Cochrane Review. In: *The Cochrane Library*, Issue 2 2003. Oxford: Update Software.

Hofmeyr GJ, Kulier R. External cephalic version for breech presentation at term. Cochrane Review. In: *The Cochrane Library*, Issue 2, 2003. Oxford: Update Software.

The circumcised woman

Larsen U, Okonofua FE. Female circumcision and obstetric complications. *Int J Gynaecol Obstet*. 2002; **77**: 255–65.

Royal College of Midwives. Female Genital Mutilation (Female Circumcision). Position Paper no. 21. London: Royal College of Midwives, 1998.

Royal College of Obstetricians and Gynaecologists. Female Genital Mutilation. Statement no. 3. London: Royal College of Obstetricians and Gynaecologists, 2003.

Perineal tear

Fitzpatrick M, Behan M, OConnell PR, O'Herlihy C. A randomised clinical trial comparing primary overlap with approximation repair of third degree tear. *Am J Obstet Gynecol* 2000; **183**: 1220–24.

Keighley MRB, Radley S, Johanson R. Consensus on prevention and management of post-obstetric bowel incontinence and third degree tear. *Clin Risk* 2000; **6**: 231–7.

Kettle C, Johanson RB. Absorbable synthetic versus catgut suture material for perineal repair. Cochrane Review. In: *The Cochrane Library*, Issue 2, 2003. Oxford: Update Software.

Kettle C, Johanson RB. Continuous versus interrupted sutures for perineal repair. Cochrane Review. In: *The Cochrane Library*, Issue 2, 2003. Oxford: Update Software.

Royal College of Obstetricians and Gynaecologists. Methods and Materials used in Perineal Repair. Clinical Green Top Guideline no. 23. London: Royal College of Obstetricians and Gynaecologists, 2000.

Sultan AH, Monga AK, Kumar D, Stanton SL. Primary repair of obstetric anal sphincter rupture using the overlap technique. *Br J Obstet Gynaecol* 1999; **106**: 318–23.

Heart disease in labour

American College of Obstetricians and Gynaecologists. Cardiac Disease in Pregnancy. Technical Bulletin no. 168. Washington, DC: American College of Obstetricians and Gynaecologists, 1992.

De Swiet M. Cardiac disease. In: Lewis G (ed). *Why Mothers Die 1997–1999. The Fifth Report of the Confidential Enquiries into Maternal Deaths in the United Kingdom*. London: RCOG Press, 2001.

Endocarditis Working group of the British Society for Antimicrobial Chemotherapy. Antibiotic prophylaxis of infective endocarditis *Lancet* 1990; **335**: 88–90.

Nelson-Piercy C. Heart disease. In: *Handbook of Obstetric Medicine*, 2nd edn. London: Martin Dunitz, 2002, pp. 22–39.

Peripartum cardiomyopathy

Mehta NJ, Mehta RN, Khan IA. Peripartum cardiomyopathy: clinical and therapeutic aspects. *Angiology* 2001; **52**: 759–62.

Olagundoye VV, Seow Y, Ashworth MA. Peripartum cardiomyopathy: a forgotten diagnosis? *Hosp Med* 2003; **64**: 50–51.

Pearson GD, Veille JC, Rahimtoola S, *et al*. Peripartum cardiomyopathy: National Heart, Lung and Blood Institute and Office of Rare Diseases (National Institutes of Health) workshop recommendations and review. *J Am Med Assoc* 2000; **283**: 1183–8.

Pre-eclampsia

Brodie H, Malinow AM. Anaesthetic management of preeclampsia/eclampsia. *Int J Obstet Anesth* 1999; **8**: 110–24.

Chappell LC, Poulton L, Halligan A, Shennan AH. Lack of consistency in research papers over the definition of pre-eclampsia. *Br J Obstet Gynaecol* 1999; **106**: 983–5.

Department of Health. *Why Mothers Die. Report of the Confidential Enquiries into Maternal Deaths in the UK, 1994–96*. London: The Stationery Office, 1998.

Duley L, Guhmezoglu AM, Henderson-Smart DT. Magnesium sulphate and other anticoagulants for women with pre-eclampsia. Cochrane Review. In: *The Cochrane Library*, Issue 2, 2003. Oxford: Update Software.

Fay TN. *Labour Ward Rules*. London: BMJ Books, 2001, p. 114.

Hasan MA, Thomas TA, Prys-Roberts C. Comparison of automatic oscillometric arterial pressure measurement with conventional auscultatory measurement in the labour ward. *Br J Anaesth* 1993; **70**: 141–4.

Idama TO, Lindlow SW. Magnesium sulphate: a review of clinical pharmacology applied to obstetrics. *Br J Obstet Gynaecol* 1998; **105**: 260–68.

Mabie WC, Gonzalez AR, Sibai BM, Amon E. A comparative trial of labetalol and hydrallazine in the acute management of severe hypertension complicating pregnancy. *Obstet Gynecol* 1987; **70**: 328–33.

Magee LA, Cham C, Waterman EJ *et al*. Hydralazine for treatment of severe hypertension in pregnancy: meta-analysis. *BMJ* 2003; **327**: 955–64.

Mortl MG, Schneider MC. Key issues in assessing, managing and treating patients presenting with severe preeclampsia. *Int J Obstet Anesth* 2000; **9**: 39–44.

National High Blood Pressure Education Program: Working Group Report on High Blood Pressure in Pregnancy. *Am J Obstet Gynecol* 2000; **183**: S1–22.

Nielson JP. Hypertensive diseases of pregnancy. In: Lewis G (ed). *Why Mothers Die 1997–99. The Fifth Report of the Confidential Enquiries into Maternal Deaths in the United Kingdom*. London: RCOG Press, 2001.

Quinn M. Automated blood pressure measurement devices: a potential source of morbidity in preeclampsia? *Am J Obstet Gynecol* 1994; **170**: 1303–7.

Ramanathan J, Bennet K. Pre-eclampsia: fluids, drugs and anaesthetic management. *Anesthesiol Clin North Am* 2003; **21**: 145–63.

Reinders A, Cuckson AC, Jones CR, *et al.* Validation of the Welch Allyn 'Vital Signs' blood pressure measurement device in pregnancy and pre-eclampsia. *Br J Obstet Gynaecol* 2003; **110**: 134–8.

Robson SC, Pearson JF. Fluid restriction policies in preeclampsia are obsolete. *Int J Obstet Anesth* 1999; **8**: 49–55.

Waisman GD, Mayorga LM, Camera MI *et al.* Magnesium plus nifedipine: potentiation od hypotensive effect in pre-eclampsia? *Am J Obstet Gynecol* 1988; **159**: 308–9.

Witlin AG, Sibai BM. Magnesium sulfate therapy in pre-eclampsia and eclampsia. *Obstet Gynecol* 1998; **92**: 883–9.

Eclampsia

Duley L, Carroli G, Belizan J *et al.* Which anticonvulsant for women with eclampsia – evidence from the collaborative eclampsia trial. *Lancet* 1995; **345**: 1455–63.

Duley L, Henderson-Smart D. Magnesium sulphate versus diazepam for eclampsia. Cochrane Review. In: *The Cochrane Library*, Issue 2, 2003. Oxford: Update Software.

Royal College of Obstetricians and Gynaecologists. Management of Eclampsia. Clinical Green Top Guideline no. 10. London: Royal College of Obstetricians and Gynaecologists, 1999.

Diabetes mellitus

Chauhan SP, Perry KG Jr. Management of diabetic ketoacidosis in the obstetric patient. *Obstet Gynecol Clin North Am* 1995; **22**: 143–55.

Diabetes UK. *Recommendations for the Management of Pregnant Women with Diabetes (Including Gestational Diabetes)*. London: Diabetes UK, 2003.

Hadden DR, McCance DR. Advances in management of type 1 diabetes and pregnancy. *Curr Opin Obstet Gynecol* 1999; **11**: 557–62.

Lean ME, Pearson DW, Sutherland HW. Insulin management during labour and delivery in mothers with diabetes. *Diabet Med* 1990; **7**: 162–4.

Epilepsy

Katz JM, Devinsky O. Primary generalized epilepsy: a risk factor for seizures in labor and delivery? *Seizure* 2003; **12**: 217–19.

Pennell PB. Pregnancy in the woman with epilepsy: maternal and fetal outcomes. *Semin Neurol* 2002; **22**: 299–308.

Scottish Obstetric Guidelines and Audit Project. *The Management of Pregnancy In Women with Epilepsy. A Clinical Practice Guideline for Professionals Involved in Maternity Care*. Aberdeen: Scottish Programme for Clinical Effectiveness in Reproductive Health, 1997.

The Royal College of Midwives. The care of women with epilepsy – guidelines for midwives. London: Royal College of Midwives 1997.

Systemic lupus erythematosus

Buchanan NMM, Khamashta MA, Kerslake S, *et al.* Practical management of pregnancy in systemic lupus erythematosus. *Fet Mat Med Rev* 1993; **5**: 223–30.

Georgiou PE, Politi EN, Katsimbri P, *et al.* Outcome of lupus pregnancy: a controlled study. *Rheumatology (Oxford)* 2000; **39**: 1014–19.

Mascola MA, Repke JT. Obstetric management of the high-risk lupus pregnancy. *Rheum Dis Clin North Am* 1997; **23**: 119–32.

Mok CC, Wong RW. Pregnancy in systemic lupus erythematosus. *Postgrad Med J* 2001; **77**: 157–65.

Other connective tissue disorders

Abouleish E. Obstetric anaesthesia and Ehlers–Danlos syndrome. *Br J Anaesth* 1980; **52**: 1283–6.

Lipscomb KJ, Clayton-Smith J, Clarke B, *et al*. Outcome of pregnancy in women with Marfan's syndrome. *Br J Obstet Gynaecol* 1997; **104**: 201–4.

Roop KA, Brost BC. Abnormal presentation in labor and fetal growth of affected infants with type III Ehlers–Danlos syndrome. *Am J Obstet Gynecol* 1999; **181**: 752–3.

Stone S, Nelson-Piercy C. Connective tissue diseases in pregnancy. *Contemp Clin Gynecol Obstet* 2001; **1**: 69–81.

The Rhesus-negative woman

Crowther C, Middleton P. Anti-D administration after childbirth for preventing Rhesus alloimmmunisation. Cochrane Review. In: *The Cochrane Library*, Issue 3, 2002. Oxford: Update Software.

Royal College of Obstetricians and Gynaecologists. Use of Anti-D Immunoglobulin for Rhesus Prophylaxis. Clinical Green Top Guideline no. 22. London: Royal College of Obstetricians and Gynaecologists, 2002.

Thromboembolism prophylaxis

Department of Health. *Why Mothers Die. Report of the Confidential Enquiries into Maternal Deaths in the UK 1994–96*. London: The Stationery Office, 1998.

Nelson-Piercy C, Obstetric thromboprophylaxis. *Br J Hosp Med* 1996; **55**: 404–8.

Acute venous thromboembolism and pulmonary embolism

Checketts MR, Wildsmith JA. Central nerve block and thromboprophylaxis – Is there a problem? *Br J Anaesth* 1999; **82**: 164–7.

Greer I. Treatment of venous thromboembolism in pregnancy. *Reprod Vasc Med* 2001; **1**: 114–19.

Horlocker TT, Wedel DJ. Spinal and epidural blockade and peri-operative low molecular weight heparin: smooth sailing on the Titanic. *Anesth Analg* 1998; **86**: 1153–6.

Royal College of Obstetricians and Gynaecologists. Thromboembolic Disease in Pregnancy and the Puerperium: Acute Management. Clinical Green Top Guideline no. 28. London: Royal College of Obstetricians and Gynaecologists, 2001.

Major haemoglobinopathy

Danzer BI, Birnbach DJ, Thys DM. Anaesthesia for the parturient with sickle cell disease. *J Clin Anaesth* 1996; **8**: 598–602.

Howard RJ. Management of sickling conditions in pregnancy. *Br J Hosp Med* 1996; **56**: 7–10.

Howard RJ, Tuck SM. Sickle cell disease and pregnancy. *Curr Obstet Gynaecol* 1995; **5**; 36–40.

Rust OA, Perry KG, Jr. Pregnancy complicated by sickle haemoglobinopathy. *Clin Obstet Gynaecol* 1995; **38**: 472–84.

Inherited coagulation disorders: haemophilia and von Willebrand disease

Conti M, Mari D, Conti E, et al. Pregnancy in women with different types of von Willebrand disease. *Obstet Gynecol* 1986; **68**: 282–5.

Kadir RA. Women and inherited bleeding disorders: pregnancy and delivery. *Semin Hematol* 1999; **36**(3 suppl 4): 28–35.

Kadir RA, Economides DL, Braithwaite J, *et al*. The obstetric experience of carriers of haemophilia. *Br J Obstet Gynaecol* 1997; **104**: 803–10.

Kadir RA, Lee CA, Sabin CA, et al. Pregnancy in women with von Willebrand's disease or factor XI deficiency. *Br J Obstet Gynaecol* 1998; **105**: 314–21.

Walker ID, Walker JJ, Colvin BT, *et al*. Investigation and management of haemorrhagic disorders in pregnancy. Haemostasis and Thrombosis Task Force. *J Clin Pathol* 1994; **47**: 100–108.

Gestational thrombocytopenia

Aster RH. 'Gestational' thrombocytopenia: a plea for conservative management. *N Engl J Med* 1990; **323**: 264–6.

Immune thrombocytopenic purpura

Kadir RA, Economides DL, Braithwaite J, *et al*. The obstetric experience of carriers of haemophilia. *Br J Obstet Gynaecol* 1997; **104**: 803–10.

Kadir RA, Lee CA, Sabin CA, *et al*. Pregnancy in women with von Willebrand's disease or factor XI deficiency. *Br J Obstet Gynaecol* 1998; **105**: 314–21.

Letsky EA. Haemostasis and epidural anaesthesia. *Int J Obstet Anaesth* 1991; **1**: 51–4.

Letsky EA, Greaves M. Guidelines on the investigation and management of thrombocytopoenia in pregnancy and neonatal alloimmune thrombocytopoenia. *Br J Haematol* 1996; **95**: 21–6.

Thrombophilia

Walker ID. Inherited coagulation disorders and thrombophilia in pregnancy. In: Bonnar J (ed.). *Recent Advances in Obstetrics and Gynaecology*, no. 20. Edinburgh: Churchill Livingstone, 1998.

Walker ID. Management of thrombophilia in pregnancy. *Blood Rev* 1991; **5**: 227–33.

Major placenta praevia

Penna LK, Pearce JM. Placenta praevia. In: Studd J (ed). *Progress in Obstetrics and Gynaecology*, vol. 11. Edinburgh: Churchill Livingstone, 1994.

Royal College of Obstetricians and Gynaecologists. Placenta Praevia: Diagnosis and Management. Clinical Green Top Guideline no. 27. London: Royal College of Obstetricians and Gynaecologists, 2001.

Sunna E, Ziadeh S. Transvaginal and transabdominal ultrasound for the diagnosis of placenta praevia. *J Obstet Gynaecol* 1999; **19**: 152–4.

Retained placenta

Carroli G, Bergel E. Umbilical vein injection for the management of retained placenta. Cochrane Review. In: *The Cochrane Library*, Issue 2, 2003. Oxford: Update Software.

Postpartum haemorrhage

American Academy of Family Physicians. *Advanced Life Support in Obstetrics (ALSO) Course Syllabus*, 4th edn. Kansas; American Academy of Family Physicians, 2000.

Drife J. Management of primary postpartum haemorrhage. *Br J Obstet Gynaecol* 1997; **104**: 275–7.

Lewis G. *Why Mothers Die 1997–1999. The Fifth Report of the Confidential Enquiries into Maternal Deaths in the United Kingdom*. London: RCOG Press, 2001.

Wilkinson C, Enkin MW. Manual removal of placenta at caesarean section. Cochrane Review. In: *The Cochrane Library*, Issue 3, 2002. Oxford: Update Software.

Disseminated intravascular coagulopathy

Toh CH, Dennis M. Disseminated intravascular coagulation: old disease, new hope. *BMJ* 2003, **327**: 974–7.

Delivery of woman at known risk of haemorrhage

Hall MH. Haemorrhage. In: Lewis G (ed). *Why Mothers Die 1997–99. The Fifth Report of the Confidential Enquiries into Maternal Deaths in the United Kingdom*. London: RCOG Press, 2001, pp 94–103.

Management of the woman who declines blood transfusion

Bonakdar MI, Eckhous AW, Backer BJ, *et al*. Major gynaecologic and obstetric surgery in Jehovah's Witnesses. *Obstet Gynaecol* 1982; **60**: 587–90.

Buscuttil D, Copplestone A. Management of blood loss in Jehovah's Witness. *Br Med J* 1995; **311**: 1115–16.

Hibbard BM *et al*. The treatment of obstetric haemorrhage in women who refuse blood transfusion. In: *Report on Confidential Enquiries into Maternal Deaths in the United Kingdom 1991–93*. London: HMSO, 1996, pp. 44–7.

Mann CM, Votto J, Kambe J, McNamee MJ. Management of the severely anaemic patient who refuses transfusion: lessons learned during the care of a Jehovah's Witness. *Ann Intern Med* 1992; **177**: 1042–8.

Reid MF, Nohn R, Birks RJS. Eclampsia and haemorrhage in a Jehovah's Witness. *Anaesthesia* 1986; **41**: 324–5.

Thomas JM. The world wide need for education in nonblood management in obstetrics and gynaecology. *J Soc Obstet Gynaecol Can* 1994; **16**: 1482–7.

Prophylactic antibiotics

British Society for Antimicrobial Chemotherapy. Endocarditis Working Party. Antibiotic prophylaxis of infective endocarditis. *Lancet* 1997; **350**: 1100.

Hopkins L, Smaill F. Antibiotic prophylaxis regimens and drugs for cesarean section. Cochrane Review. In: *The Cochrane Library*, Issue 2, 2003. Oxford: Update Software.

PHLS Group B Streptococcus Working Group. Interim 'best practice' recommendations for the prevention of neonatal group B streptococcal infection in the UK. London: Central Public Health Laboratory, 2000.

Intrapartum pyrexia

Thompson W. Genital tract sepsis. In: Lewis G (ed). *Why Mothers Die, 1997–99. The Fifth Report of the Confidential Enquiries into Maternal Deaths in the United Kingdom*. London: RCOG Press, 2001, pp. 121–9.

Intrapartum antibiotic prophylaxis for group B *Streptococcus*

American Academy of Pediatrics. Revised guidelines for prevention of early-onset group B streptococcal disease. *Pediatrics* 1997; **99**: 489–96.

Centers for Disease Control. Prevention of perinatal group B streptococcal disease: a public health perspective. *Morb Mortal Wkly Rep* 1996; **45** (RR-7): 1–20.

PHLS Group B Streptococcus Working Group. Interim 'best practice' recommendations for the prevention of neonatal group B streptococcal infection in the UK. London: Central Public Health Laboratory, 2000.

Royal College of Obstetricians and Gynaecologists. Prevention of Early Onset Neonatal Group B Streptococcal Disease. Draft guideline. London: Royal College of Obstetricians and Gynaecologists, 2003.

Smaill F. Intrapartum antibiotics for group B streptococcal colonisation. Cochrane Review. In: *The Cochrane Library*, Issue 2, 2003. Oxford: Update Software.

Genital herpes

McLean A, Regan L, Carrington D. *Infection and Pregnancy. Report of an RCOG Study Group*. London: RCOG Press, 2001.

Royal College of Obstetricians and Gynaecologists. Management of Genital Herpes in Pregnancy. Clinical Green Top Guideline no. 30. London: Royal College of Obstetricians and Gynaecologists, 2002.

Smith JR, Cowan FM, Munday P. The management of herpes simplex virus infections in pregnancy. *Br J Obstet Gynaecol* 1998; **105**: 255–60.

Human immunodeficiency virus

British HIV Association. Guidelines for the management of HIV infection in pregnant women and the prevention of mother-to-child transmission. *HIV Med* 2001; **2**: 314–34.

Irish Infection Society. National guidelines for the active management of HIV in pregnancy. *Ir Med J* 2001; **94**: 137–40.

Kuczkowski KM. Human immunodeficiency virus in the parturient. *J Clin Anesth* 2003; **15**: 224–33.

Minkoff H. Human immunodeficiency virus infection in pregnancy. *Obstet Gynecol* 2003; **101**: 797–810.

Public Health Service Task Force Perinatal HIV Guidelines Working Group. Summary of the updated recommendation from the Public Health Service Task Force to reduce perinatal human immunodeficiency virus-1 transmission in the United States. *Obstet Gynaecol* 2002; **99**: 1117–26. Full report downloadable from www.aidsinfo.org.

Royal College of Midwives. HIV and AIDS. Position paper 16a. London: Royal College of Midwives, 1998.

Rupture of the uterus

Clements RV. Operative obstetrics. In: Clements RV (ed). *Risk Management and Litigation in Obstetrics and Gynaecology*. London: Royal Society of Medicine Press, 2001, pp. 238–40.

Cervical tear and paravaginal haematoma

Ridgway LE. Puerperal emergency: vaginal and vulval haematoma. *Obstet Gynecol Clin North Am* 1995; **22**: 275–82.

Sheikh GN. Perinatal genital haematomas. *Obstet Gynecol* 1971; **38**: 571–5.

Shoulder dystocia

American Academy of Family Physicians. *Advanced Life Support in Obstetrics (ALSO) Course Syllabus*, 4th edn. Kansas: American Academy of Family Physicians 2000.

Johnstone FD, Myerscough PR. Shoulder dystocia. *Br J Obstet Gynaecol* 1998; **105**: 811–15.
Owen P, Bain C. Shoulder dystocia. *Hosp Med* 1998; **59**: 698–703.
Pearson JF. Shoulder dystocia. *Curr Obstet Gynaecol* 1996; **6**: 30–34.

Inverted uterus

Irani S, Jordan J. Management of uterine inversion. *Curr Obstet Gynaecol* 1997; **7**: 232–5.
Johnson NP, Bishop E, Buist R. Hydrostatic replacement of acute inversion of the uterus can cause acute pulmonary oedema by intrauterine fluid intravasation. *J Obstet Gynaecol* 1999; **19**: 544–5.
Ogueh O, Ayida G. Acute uterine inversion: a new technique of hydrostatic replacement. *Br J Obstet Gynaecol* 1997; **104**: 951–2.
Rachagan SP, Sivanesratnam V, Kok KP, Raman S. Acute puerperal inversion of the uterus – an obstetric emergency. *Aust NZ J Obstet Gynaecol* 1988; **28**: 29–32.

Amniotic fluid embolism

Clark SL, Hankins GDV, Dudley DA *et al.* Amniotic fluid embolism: analysis of the national registry. *Am J Obstet Gynecol* 1995; **172**: 1158–69.
Howell P, Amniotic fluid embolism. In: Collis R, Plaat F, Urquhart J (eds). *Textbook of Obstetric Anaesthesia.* London: Greenwich Medical Media, 2002, Chapter 17, pp. 263–89.

Sudden maternal collapse

Advanced Life Support Working Group of the European Resuscitation Council. The 1998 European Resuscitation Council guidelines for adult advanced life support. *Br Med J* 1998; **316**: 1863–9.
Hayashi RH. Obstetric collapse. In: Kean L, Baker PN, Edelstone DI (eds). *Best Practice in Labour Ward Management.* Edinburgh: WB Saunders, 2000.

Latex allergy

Adeley J, Rowland A. Managing the risk of latex allergy in healthcare workers and patients. *Clin Risk* 1999; **5**: 129–31.
Diaz T, Martinez T, Antepara I, *et al.* Latex allergy as a risk during delivery. *Br J Obstet Gynaecol* 1996; **103**: 173–5.
Eckhout GV, Jr, Ayad S. Anaphylaxis due to airborne exposure to latex in a primigravida. *Anesthesiology* 2001; **4**: 1034–5.
Santos R, Hernandez-Ayup S, Galache P, *et al.* Severe latex allergy after a vaginal examination during labour: a case report. *Am J Obstet Gynecol* 1997; **177**: 1543–4.
Shingai Y, Nakagawa K, Kato T, *et al.* Severe allergy in a pregnant woman after vaginal examination with a latex glove. *Gynecol Obstet Invest* 2002; **54**: 183–4.

Anaphylaxis

British Medical Association and Royal Pharmaceutical Society of Great Britain. *British National Formulary*, no. 43. London: British Medical Association and Royal Pharmaceutical Society of Great Britain, 2002, p. 156.

Mid-trimester termination of pregnancy for fetal abnormality

Royal College of Obstetricians and Gynaecologists. *Termination of Pregnancy for Fetal Abnormality.* London: RCOG, 1996.

Appendix I: Guidance for obtaining consent to treatment

Every adult woman of sound mind has a right to determine what can be done with her own body. She has an absolute right to refuse to consent to treatment for any reason, rational or irrational, or for no reason at all, even where the decision may lead to her own death. A healthcare provider who treats a woman without her consent could be liable in negligence or in the crime of battery. In the context of the guidance below, 'treatment' includes diagnostic procedures.

Good practice requires the provider to ensure that the patient understands what is proposed and consents to it, before proceeding with treatment or investigation. Where some form of consent has been given, it is important not to exceed the consent given or to carry out a procedure unrelated to the consent.

Who gives consent?

No one can legally give consent on behalf of an adult of sound mind. A spouse or other relative may not give consent or withhold consent if the woman is competent.

How valid is a consent?

The following are necessary for a consent to be valid:

- patient must have the mental capacity to make the decision
- patient must make the decision without undue influence
- patient must be given sufficient information about the treatment.

If there is any doubt about the competence of a patient, then the consultant should be informed. Guidance can be obtained from *Assessment of Mental Capacity – Guidance for Doctors and Lawyers* (see Further reading, p. 230). In some cases it might be necessary to seek a court declaration.

Consent should not be obtained under duress. Where there is a recognized undue influence, this should be reported to the supervising consultant or senior midwife.

The professional obtaining consent should declare any potential conflict of interest.

The patient should be given sufficient time to consider the information given. For elective procedures, a reasonable interval should elapse between obtaining consent and performing treatment.

How much information should be given?

This is generally a matter of clinical judgement depending on individual needs and the complexity of treatment; but enough information should be given to ensure that the patient understands:

- the nature of the treatment
- the benefits of the treatment
- the consequences of the treatment and of refusal of treatment
- any substantial risk of the treatment.

Where there are alternatives, these should be discussed and reasons should be given for recommending a particular option. Oral information should be supplemented with information leaflets wherever possible. The use of such leaflets should be recorded.

Who should obtain consent?

To ensure that the patient is informed fully, it is important that her consent is obtained by the person who will provide the treatment. However, this task may be delegated to any professional who:

- is suitably trained and competent
- has sufficient knowledge of the proposed treatment
- understands the risks involved
- has access to an appropriate support person.

The person providing the treatment remains responsible for ensuring that a meaningful consent has been given.

When is a written consent required?

Express (as opposed to implied) consent may be oral or written. An oral consent is as valid as a written consent, but written consent provides documentary evidence that a discussion took place.

Where oral consent has been obtained, it should be documented in the notes. This should be sufficient for most non-invasive procedures.

Written consent should be obtained for any procedure or treatment carrying any substantial risk or substantial side-effect.

 Short-hand and abbreviations should not be used and alterations to the consent form should be avoided.

Special cases

- A minor under 16 can give consent if she is Fraser (Gillick) competent.
- An official link worker should be used if the patient does not speak English.
- Special arrangements must be made for patients with hearing or speech disabilities.

Procedures for which written consent should be obtained

- All gynaecological and obstetric procedures performed in theatre under local or general anaesthesia.
- Amniocentesis.
- Licensed infertility treatment.
- Medical termination of pregnancy.

Procedures for which verbal consent should be obtained and documented

- Blood transfusion.
- Induction of labour.
- Vaginal examination in labour.
- Rectal examination.
- Vaginal examination by medical student.
- Amniotomy (artificial rupture of fetal membranes).
- Breech vaginal delivery.
- Instrumental delivery.
- Administration of vitamin K injection to baby.
- External cephalic version.
- Fetal scalp blood sampling.
- Epidural analgesia.
- Administration of enema/suppository.
- Application of fetal scalp electrode.
- Administration of anti-D immunoglobulin.
- Syntometrine injection.
- Episiotomy.
- Repair of episiotomy.
- Pipelle endometrial sampling.
- Gonadotrophin induction of ovulation.
- Insertion of oestradiol implant.
- Administration of gonadotrophin-releasing hormone analogue.
- Colposcopy/treatment to the cervix.
- Paracentesis abdominis.
- Insertion/removal of intrauterine contraceptive device (IUCD).

Further reading

British Medical Association and Law Society. *Assessment of Mental Capacity – Guidance for Doctors and Lawyers*. London: British Medical Association and Law Society, 1995.

Department of Health. *A Guide to Consent for Examination or Treatment*. www.doh.gov.uk/consent

General Medical Council. *Seeking Patients' Consent: the Ethical Considerations*. London: General Medical Council, 1999.

Appendix II: Standards for administering blood transfusion

Background

Despite improvements in the safety of blood transfusion, errors still occur, sometimes resulting in fatality. Errors commonly arise from incorrect labelling of a blood sample, laboratory mistakes or administering the blood product to the wrong patient. Most of the errors occur not in emergency intraoperative situations, but on the wards.

In the first two years (1996–98) of voluntary reporting of serious hazards of blood transfusion in the UK and Ireland (the SHOT initiative), 366 cases were reported. Of these, 191 (52%) were 'wrong blood to patient' episodes. Analysis revealed multiple errors of identification. In 1999/2000, 'wrong blood' incidents (201 cases) accounted for 69% of all reported incidents. Wrong blood incidents are, without exception, avoidable errors.

In the first four years of the SHOT initiative, there were eight reported deaths and 54 cases of major morbidity associated with ABO-incompatible transfusions. There were 16 cases of potential Rhesus D sensitization in young female patients.

In many cases, there was a sequence of errors (in one case, there were seven errors).

The single most important error resulting in mis-transfusion is failure of the bedside checking procedure immediately before administering the transfusion. In the first two years of SHOT, the bedside check failed to detect discrepancy in blood or patient identity in a total of 80 cases, despite being carried out by two people (one always a qualified nurse or doctor). In 20 incidents, the patient had no identity wristband.

This guidance is written to inform the training and practice of staff on the maternity unit, with a view to preventing errors in the administration of blood products. It is included in the induction of new staff and should be read in conjunction with the Trust policy on blood transfusion.

Indications and techniques of blood transfusion are outside the scope of this appendix,

Obtaining consent

Except in emergencies or unconscious patients, the purpose, benefits and risks of blood transfusion should be explained to the patient. The alternatives to transfusion and the implications of declining a transfusion should also be discussed.

This discussion, and the patient's verbal consent to blood transfusion, should be documented.

The patient should be given the information leaflet *Your Questions about Blood Transfusion Answered* (see Further reading, p. 233).

Collecting a specimen for group-and-save/cross-match

The labels and cards must be completed *at the patient's bedside*, with the case notes available for reference.

Do not use pre-labelled bottles. First obtain the blood specimen, then label the bottles at the bedside.

The blood specimen should not be obtained from an arm being used for infusion of IV fluids.

When the doctor signs the request form, he or she is confirming that the sample is identified correctly.

Previous transfusion records should be consulted.

An IV cannula should be sited before the cross-matched blood is sent for.

Checking procedure for blood transfusion

Ensure that *this* blood product is for *this* patient:

■ Before transfusion, the labelling on the blood product must be checked against specific patient-identification details. This check must be carried out by two members of staff, one of whom must be a registered nurse or midwife.
■ Read the wristband and check that this corresponds with the label on the blood product. Errors with wristbands may occur, so if the patient is conscious, ask her to state her forename, family name and date of birth.
■ If there are any discrepancies in spelling or identification number, transfusion should be withheld and the blood transfusion department contacted immediately.
■ Check records of any previous blood grouping against the current report.
■ There are two labels on the blood product bag, indicating:
  – name of patient
  – hospital number
  – patient's blood group
  – donor unit number
  – compatibility type
  – donor's blood group
  – date and time of transfusion.

- These details must be checked against the form sent with the blood from the blood bank, and signed. One label must be removed and put in the patient's records.
- The final bedside check provides an important opportunity to detect errors that may have been made earlier in the process of requesting blood.

Documentation

The following should be entered in the case notes:

- consent (verbal will suffice)
- details of all blood products transfused (as above)
- time transfusion commenced and ended
- observations, including pulse rate and temperature
- any transfusion reactions.

Errors should be documented and reported as prescribed in the Trust's policy on significant event reporting.

Further reading

McClelland DBL (ed). *Handbook of Transfusion Medicine*, 3rd edn. London: The Stationery Office 2001.

National Blood Service. *Your Questions about Blood Transfusion Answered* (an information leaflet). National Blood Service, 2001.

Serious Hazards of Transfusion, Annual Report 1999/2000. Manchester; SHOT Steering Group, March 2001. Accessible at www.shot.demon.co.uk

Szama K. 355 reports of transfusion-associated deaths. *Transfusion* 1990; **30**: 583.

Szama K. Practical issues in informed consent for blood transfusion. *Am J Clin Pathol* 1997; **107**: S72–4.

Williams FG. Consent for transfusion. A duty of care. *Br Med J* 1997; **315**: 380–81.

Williamson LM, Lowe S, Love EM, *et al.* Serious hazards of transfusion (SHOT) initiative: analysis of the first two annual reports. *Br Med J* 1999; **319**: 16–19.

Glossary of terms

Abnormal lie	Any lie other than longitudinal
Advance directive	A declaration by a competent person stating what should happen if they lose the capacity to make decisions for themselves
Chorionicity	Number of placentas in multiple pregnancy – single shared placenta or one each
Cleidotomy	Intentional fracture of the baby's collar bone, to facilitate delivery
Clotting (or coagulation) profile	This would usually comprise prothrombin time, activated partial thromboplastin time, fibrinogen and fibrinogen degradation products
D-dimer	A protein that is released into the circulation during the process of fibrin blood clot breakdown. D-dimer present in circulation is used as an indicator of a blood clot being formed and broken down somewhere in the body. D-dimer levels in pregnancy are higher than in the non-pregnant state
Dystocia	Dysfunctional labour
Falx cerebri	Structure formed by two leaves of dura, along the sagittal suture
Fifths palpable	The number of fifths of the baby's head palpable above the pelvic brim. This corresponds with the number of finger breadths palpable above the symphysis pubis. When the head is 'engaged', the bony presenting part (ie caput excluded) is at the level of the ischial spines, and the baby's head is 1/5 to 2/5 palpable abdominally
Hydrops fetalis	Condition characterized by generalized oedema, often with ascites, pleural effusion and pericardial effusion
Instrumental delivery	Ventouse or forceps delivery
Ischial spines	Bony landmark in pelvis; used to express level of descent of the baby's head

Malpresentation	Abnormal presentation – any presentation other than cephalic
Partogram	Graphic documentation of events in labour
Patient Group Direction	A document that allows a registered healthcare professional (normally a nurse or midwife) to supply or administer a prescription-only medicine to a patient without the drug having been prescribed by a doctor
Plasma substitute	Infusion used to expand and maintain blood volume. Gelofusine and Haemaccel are gelatine of bovine origin. They are recommended in this book as they have no effect on haemostasis. Maize starch products (such as Hespan) and hydrolysed starch (Dextran) inhibit clotting
Rhesus isoimmunization	Condition arising from incompatibility of Rhesus blood groups in mother and baby
Rule 42 (of the UKCC)	Miwives have a **statutory** duty to keep good records: 'A practising midwife shall keep as contemporaneously as is reasonable detailed records of observations, care given and medicine or other forms of pain relief administered by her to all mothers and babies' 42(1); 'A midwife must not destroy or arrange for the destruction of official records which have been made whilst she is in professional attendance upon a case ...' 42(3)
Tocolysis	Therapeutic arrest of uterine contractions
Tocolytic	Drug used to stop uterine contractions
Ventouse delivery	Delivery by vacuum extraction

Index